expecting wonder

EXPECTING WONDER
The Transformative Experience
of Becoming a Mother

Published in association with Books & Such Literary
Management, 52 Mission Circle (Suite 122), PMB 170,
Santa Rosa, CA 95409-5370 (www.booksandsuch.com).

All Scripture quotations are from the New Living Translation,
the English Standard Version, or the Berean Study Bible.

Cover design: Lindsey Owens
Cover image: Anna Putina/istock

Print ISBN: 978-1-5064-5890-8
eBook ISBN: 978-1-5064-5891-5

expecting wonder

THE TRANSFORMATIVE EXPERIENCE OF BECOMING A MOTHER

BRITTANY L. BERGMAN

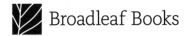 Broadleaf Books

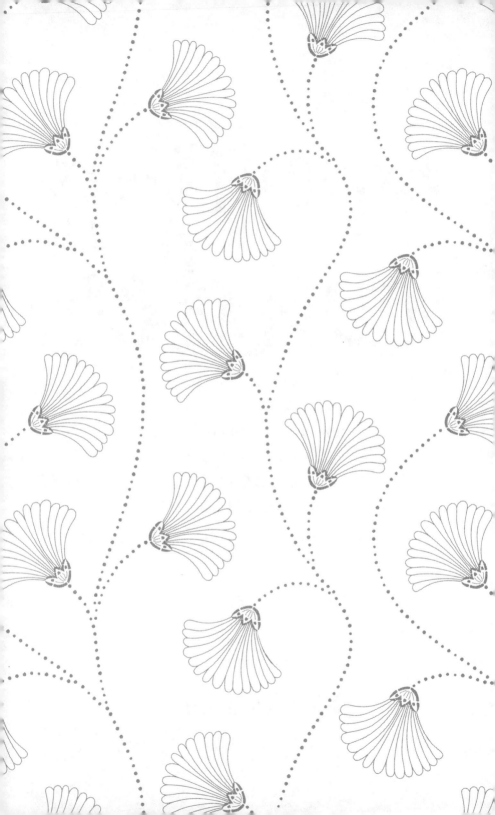

For Selah and Eamon—
being your mother is a true delight.

contents

Third Trimester
Anticipating Change and Welcoming Wonder...134

Author's Note

There are a number of films and short stories that explore what life would be like if we all lived with recording devices implanted in our bodies. The possibilities are mixed: it would be both helpful and horrifying to be able to relive each moment of our lives in perfect detail. As someone prone to overthinking every awkward thing I've said or done (and there are plenty), this sounds like my nightmare. And yet I can see the utility of such a device in writing about the past.

Since I lack access to a built-in recording device, I've reconstructed the events in this book to the best of my memory, though to spare you some boredom and confusion, I've collapsed the timeline in a few places. I've changed the names and identifying details of some people in order to respect their privacy, and I've also changed the names of a few places.

Even with these minor adjustments, this story captures real people and real events from a momentous time in my life. Though I hope this story will be widely applicable, it is uniquely my own.

Introduction

A Craving for Stories

Pregnancy is both undeniably beautiful and totally bizarre. For nine months (sometimes closer to ten!), we allow another human to take up residence inside our bodies. We literally grow a brand-new temporary organ that's responsible for feeding and protecting the baby; a pulsating cord connects the baby to that organ and to us; we experience energy depletion, cramping, stretching, emotional swings, and heartburn in the process.

Astonishing as it is, pregnancy could also be called common-place—as many as 211 million pregnancies occur every year.[1] But for those of us who have nurtured other humans inside our wombs, we know it is nothing short of miraculous: an embryo that starts out no bigger than a grain of sand will become a fully formed baby.

Pregnancy is also complicated and fraught with big emotions. The occupancy of our wombs at any given moment—full or empty—can cause sorrow or joy, grief or relief, envy or celebration.

For many new moms, and for me personally, pregnancy can be equal parts overwhelming and joyful—sometimes in the very same minute. My first pregnancy was uncomplicated medically, but even so, I wrestled with fear and uncertainty and anxiety and darkness. I wanted to be completely in control (thus, capable) of keeping this precious life safe, but I also knew that kind of responsibility would crush me. I tried to be the perfect pregnant woman because somehow I thought that would mean I'd be the perfect mom. I longed to relish every minute of the miracle happening inside my body, but I was often swept away by the to-do list instead: creating a baby registry and decorating the nursery and envisioning a birth plan and reading the books.

---

1   The World Health Report 2005: Make Every Mother and Child Count (Geneva, Switzerland: World Health Organization, 2005), 48. https://www.who.int/whr/2005/en.

Oh, the books. There is no shortage of volumes out there about pregnancy, and no shortage of expectations that expecting moms will read them and follow their rules to the letter. The irony isn't lost on me that I'm writing this in yet another book about pregnancy. But what I found was that so many of those pages approach pregnancy as a medical condition to be managed rather than as a transformation, a transition, a sacred moment in time to be savored and celebrated.

We read about what's happening to our babies each week: the fingers are forming, the head is starting to look more humanlike, the heart is beating, the lungs are developing. We read about what's to come: what labor will feel like, how we can manage the pain, the best way to breathe through the contractions, the pros and cons of getting the epidural.

Much of this information is good and helpful, but what I craved most when I was pregnant (besides donuts) were *stories*. Not more medical information, labor strategies, or lists telling me exactly what to pack in my hospital bag, but stories of women who had been there, who had felt the fear and the pain and the joy and weight of it all. Stories of women who had gained weight and felt ashamed but also empowered; stories of women who had argued with their husbands over what to hang on the nursery walls; stories of women who felt overwhelmed by the big-box baby stores and had to realize that their ability to mother well wasn't wrapped up in choosing the right swaddling blankets.

During a time that is so focused on the physical reality of growing a baby and preparing for life with that tiny person, I offer these words as a love letter to you, bearing witness to the unseen ways in which you are changing and growing and being shaped. This book is about more than the biological reality of growing a human; it's about how each moment of pregnancy shapes *us* as we become mothers.

The book you're holding is a collection of stories about how I was broken open for the sake of another and for the sake of becoming a mother. These are not stories of how God delivered me from all my fears, nor are they stories of how God was the perfect answer to every worry and question and doubt.

These are stories of how I wrestled with God, how I marveled at God's design but struggled to trust in it, how I delighted in God's goodness but didn't always believe it. These are stories of a time when I was stretched in every possible way—physically, of course, but also emotionally and mentally and spiritually. These are the stories of how my body made room for two things at once—for myself and for my baby—and how my heart did too—for fear and joy, for sorrow and delight, for feeling deeply unsettled but choosing to celebrate anyway.

Together, they are the story of how I became a mother.

There are many ways in which women become mothers, each one beautiful and significant. It is not my intention to say that pregnancy is the only way, or the most important way, or the best way. Pregnancy just so happens to be my road into motherhood. I am one woman who was pregnant at a moment in time, but through this tiny blip in human history, my identity was fundamentally transformed.

Whether you're hoping to become pregnant or trying to decide if you even want kids; whether you're pregnant for the first time or the fifth time; whether you're dealing with the pain of infertility, pregnancy loss, or an intensely difficult pregnancy; whether you're done bearing babies or just getting started, I hope this book will be a companion for you. I hope you find encouragement and solidarity here. I pray these words help you to make meaning of the transformation you're experiencing and cause you to linger in the fleeting moments of this season.

Above all, I hope you can sense me squeezing your hand, looking you in the eye, and telling you not that everything will be fine and perfect but that I'm here with you, I wholeheartedly believe you can do this, and right in this moment, you can expect wonder.

Wrestling with Fear and Embracing Mystery

1

The "Right" Reasons

I've always had a nagging sense that I'm behind. Behind my friends who knew which college they wanted to attend. Behind my class-mates who weren't changing majors after sophomore year. Behind my roommates who were getting married. Behind my peers who were making more money and buying houses and saving for retirement. Behind my friends who were having their first babies, and then their second and third.

When my husband, Dan, and I first got married, we decided that we'd wait at least two years to have a baby and that January of a new year would be the perfect time to start trying. The summer before, however, I suggested we bump the timeline up by a few months. I wouldn't have admitted it then, but I was motivated primarily by fear and comparison: most of my friends already had kids or were pregnant, and, knowing that it could take months or years to conceive, I didn't want to lose any more time. I was tired of feeling behind, and I was afraid that if we waited too long and I couldn't get pregnant, I'd lose my footing and slip so far back that there would be no catching up.

Trying to have a baby out of fear or comparison is not a great idea. In fact, I don't think making decisions out of fear or comparison is a great approach in general, but I also know how all-consuming those emotions can be and how easily they can take hold of us.

One night in September, Dan and I were sitting on our couch, my legs stretched across his lap as we debated starting another show or playing a round of cards. I took a deep breath and mentioned one more time that I'd really like to start trying for a baby in November—it was only two months from then and only two months earlier than our agreed-upon date. Surely this meet-in-the-middle idea would be acceptable to both of us.

Dan glanced over at me, concern and a touch of defensiveness in his expression. "We both agreed that January was a good time to start trying. Why are you pushing for just two months sooner?"

I made some flimsy excuse about how there didn't seem to be a need to wait that long, and wouldn't it be fun to maybe, possibly find out good news around Christmastime?

I could tell he didn't quite believe me; we'd been together long enough that he knew when I was holding something back. He prodded again: "What difference does two months really make?"

"Exactly. What difference does two months really make? Why not start trying in case it takes longer than we're expecting?"

His eyes and jaw softened as he sensed the undertone of fear in my words. This concern about not being able to get pregnant had been an ongoing conversation for us since before we got married, when I first started charting my cycles in preparation for our wedding (after which we planned to use the fertility awareness method to prevent pregnancy).

I realized after a few months of tracking my fertility that I did not have an ideal cycle for achieving pregnancy and that even if I did get pregnant, I'd still face the normal risk of miscarriage during the first trimester. I envisioned months of struggle stretching out before me, months of crying at the sight of blood that signaled an empty womb. I couldn't imagine a world in which I would get pregnant quickly, and I wanted to get a jump on the heartache and the waiting.

I explained all this to Dan, saying nothing new, nothing I had not shared before.

He told me, also saying nothing new, nothing he had not shared before, that he didn't believe we would face the heartache I was expecting—the heartache I was already putting myself through by imagining the worst. I had a less-than-ideal cycle, yes. But I was young and healthy, and so was he, and besides, Bergmans have strong swimmers. There were already eight grandchildren on his side of the family. While I usually appreciated his optimism and laughed at those kinds of silly comments, that night his words sounded like naïve faith.

"You don't understand," I said, shaking my head. "You're not the one charting my cycles. You haven't done the reading. You don't know how unlikely it is that I'll get pregnant quickly. You don't know what it feels like to be consumed by worry. And you're not the one who's going to agonize while I wait for my period every month." Tears that had been pooling behind my eyes began to trickle down my face. "It feels like you don't believe me."

Dan pulled me close, reassuring me that no, he didn't know how I felt, and no, he couldn't understand why I was worried before the thing I feared had even come to fruition. He acknowledged in a whisper that it was true, I was the one who knew far more about our chances, but even so, I was letting fear control me. He looked me in the eye and said he wasn't willing to try any sooner—not because he wasn't ready but because we wouldn't be doing it for the right reasons.

My heart sank. I knew he was right and that the conversation was over until January. Still, I felt my footing give way as I fell further behind.

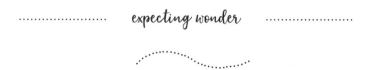

As I get older, the gaps of time between me and my friends—starting careers and getting married and having babies—seem unbelievably small, like speed bumps on a residential street. But at the time they formed, they seemed like mountains that would take ages to scale, the distance between me and the other side—the perceived greener side—nearly infinite.

Sometimes I felt ashamed for wanting to "keep up," and the platitudes I often heard from well-meaning people drifted through my head: *Don't worry so much about what other people are doing. Do what's right for you!* What I'm coming to realize is that my desire to get pregnant was only partially a competitive fear about being behind. I was also afraid of being isolated from my friends as they experienced a huge life change that I couldn't understand. It was a place I'd been before, and I didn't want to go there again.

I was enjoying being single when all my friends got married, and even though I was genuinely happy for them, it was still difficult and painful to hear them talk about the details of weddings and married life. When many of my friends started getting promoted at work, assuming roles of increased leadership and responsibility, I started over in a new career, taking an unpaid internship and waiting tables to help make ends meet. When my friends began having babies, I knew it wasn't the right time for me, but I wished I could relate to them as their lives were changing so significantly.

For the first twenty years or so of our lives, we go through roughly the same stages at the same time as our friends: moving up to the next grade level, graduating together, and making plans for college or trade schools or jobs. At that point, the path becomes less clear-cut, and we diverge—and it's in those divergences that pain and insecurity sneak in. We question whether we're doing the right thing when it looks different from what everyone else is doing.

When we've been on a preconceived path for as long as we can remember, going rogue feels risky. But the thing is, *everyone* is going rogue. There's no road map for this part of life. We get to make our own choices, forge our own paths, decide what we want and when we're ready for it. That power can be frightening at first—but when harnessed and examined, it can lead to some of the most exciting and meaningful decisions of our lives.

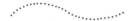

In the months after my talk with Dan, I decided to examine my reasons for wanting a baby and to cultivate joy and excitement about expanding our family.

Aside from my fears about being behind or feeling isolated, why did I want kids? And why now?

I hadn't always wanted children, but as I got deeper into adult-hood, I began to envision what I wanted my life to look like over the next ten, twenty, fifty years. When I was a kid, the future stretched out as an abstraction—a fuzzy kind of eternity called Being a Grown-Up. People constantly asked what I wanted to be when I grew up, so the only concrete thing I could picture about adulthood was my job. But as I approached this stage, the fuzziness began to recede, like dialing into a station on an old-school radio, and I could see that the grown-up years were about more than what job I might want to do. There would be decades of life to live—and I realized I didn't want to spend those decades only pursuing my career.

Of course, there were plenty of ways I could have built a fulfilling and meaningful life without children. But as I watched my friends be-come parents and saw how much they adored their kids, I began to feel pulled in the direction of motherhood.

When I was growing up, my family moved every three to four years, and in the awkward in-between phases, before we'd made new friends, my brother and sister were my closest companions. I loved playing dolls with my brother and taking care of my baby sister, who was born when I was almost nine. We spent hours running around our backyard together, building forts on precious snow-day mornings and leaping through the sprinkler on scorching summer afternoons.

In my memories, my siblings are the stars of the show, and my mother is more like the setting, a consistent backdrop to our childhood: she was always there to facilitate our activities, referee our fights, and remind us how loved we were. She took an obvious joy in motherhood, and on every first day of school she would tell us what a treat it had been to have us home with her, how much she would miss us all day, and how she couldn't wait for our next school break. Because my mom had made motherhood seem like a gift, when I thought more concretely about my future, I realized I wanted a brood of my own.

Dan grew up in a large family with four siblings, and he had always wanted kids. I had come around to the idea of children before we met, and together we dreamed of our future kids and the pieces of our childhoods we were eager to recreate with them—vacations out west to national parks; summers at his family's cottage, nestled on a lake in northern Illinois; dinners around the table, absent of proper manners but with plenty of belly laughs and conversations about our days. We love this world so deeply—the shock of mountains stretching as high and far as you can see; the melty, drippy goodness of ice cream on a hot summer day; the fiery reds and burnt oranges of a midwestern autumn; the hushed serenity of a snowfall. We wanted to experience creation all over again through the eyes of our kids.

And ultimately, having children felt like a natural extension of our love for God and our love for each other. If I couldn't get pregnant, we knew we would open our home and our hearts to children somehow—

by adopting, becoming foster parents, or some other way we couldn't imagine yet.

As I charted my cycle each month, I still feared a long journey to pregnancy. Sometimes fear got the better of me and led to moments of comparison. But thanks to the gracious honesty of my husband and some hard internal work, it became more important to me to have a baby out of true excitement, joy, and desire—not because I was afraid of falling behind.

The "right" and "wrong" reasons to have a baby aren't black and white, but if you listen to your own voice—to the mother's intuition that is already taking root—you'll discover the reasons that are right for *you*. Perhaps you grew up in a large, raucous family and want to recreate that for another generation. Perhaps you were adopted and want to provide a loving home for other children who are waiting. Perhaps you see motherhood as a chance to unleash your creativity or love or nurturing abilities. Perhaps you want kids eventually, and there's simply nothing stopping you at this moment. Perhaps when you picture the next thirty years of holidays, there are children around the table, then the partners of those grown children, and then the children of those children. Perhaps you've always dreamed of being a mom.

There's nothing that can make us fully ready for the life-altering experience of bringing a child into the world—no amount of sleep we can bank, no perfect amount of stability in our jobs, no set amount of money saved, no fixed number of years with our partners. May that realization not discourage us but free us to pursue motherhood when we decide the time is right—and to find meaning in the process.

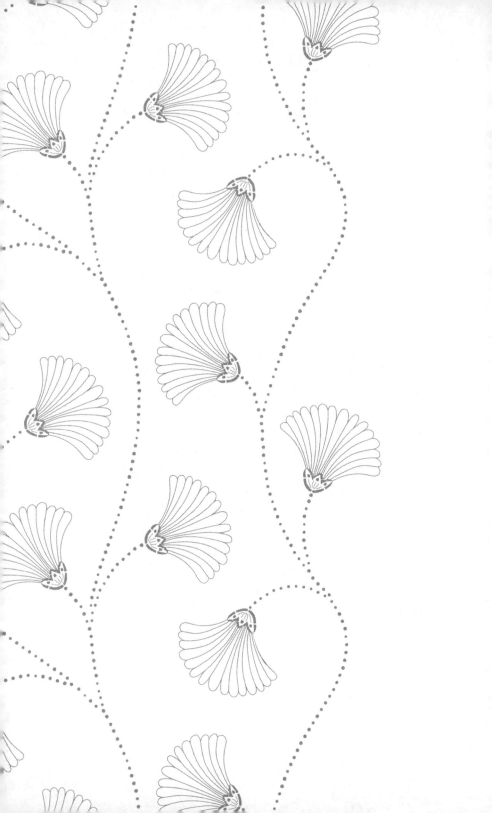

The Two-Week Wait

2

"I feel like with each passing day, I'm getting further down a road that leads to infertility rather than closer to a baby. Is that silly?"

I texted these words to my closest friend, Erin, on a gray winter day. My cubicle was several offices removed from a window, so I couldn't see the iron skies and blustery weather, but I felt them anyway. Winter in Chicago has a way of sinking into the soul. You can't shake off the dreariness like the snowflakes from your hair; it clings to and clogs up your insides, like the grimy ice stuck inside a tailpipe on a subzero day.

Perhaps the weather had something to do with my mood, but my feelings were rooted in something else too—something that wouldn't pass with a simple shift of the clouds. I was stuck in the middle of the dreaded two-week wait.

I'd been tracking my cycles for more than two years—at first to prevent pregnancy and now to try for a baby. I took my temperature every morning with an especially sensitive thermometer and checked my cervical fluid for signs of fertility. (The truly devoted even check the openness and position of the cervix.) I recorded the data on a very medical-looking chart, which helped me figure out when to have sex (or when not to, depending on the goal). More than a when-to-do-the-deed chart, this tool helped me understand my body in ways I certainly never learned in middle school sex ed. As it turned out, there was a ton of information I could glean about my body by observing the patterns of my cycle over many months.

Within the first six months of tracking, I realized my luteal phase—the second phase of the menstrual cycle, starting from the time of ovulation and lasting until the beginning of the period—was shorter than average, lasting eight to ten days instead of the typical twelve to fourteen. Because an embryo takes an average of ten to twelve days to implant, it was likely that I'd experience chemical pregnancies, passing the fertilized eggs before they had a chance to become viable. I believed this meant I would lose babies without ever knowing they existed. According to everything I'd read, it could realistically take six to twelve months to even get pregnant, and I'd be more likely than other women to miscarry.

I wish I could say I put this issue on the back burner after I discovered it, thinking something like, *That sounds like a problem for future Brittany to deal with,* or even, *I'll cross that bridge when I get there. No need to get worked up since I'm not ready to have kids yet.* But I didn't. I tend to catastrophize every perceived problem, jumping ten steps ahead to worst possible conclusion. I did the same with this: I worried about it late at night, so much so that I couldn't sleep. I stressed about how to fix it *right now*. I talked to Dan about how I didn't want to face infertility, and then I worried some more.

I took a natural supplement to boost progesterone and lengthen my luteal phase. It didn't work. I drank red raspberry leaf tea, switched to organic meat, ate more spinach, took B-complex vitamins and folate, and cut out dairy. Nothing. My cycle continued to hover in the too-short range.

So when I texted Erin that day, I was jumping to conclusions—but they were conclusions I believed were well founded and even inevitable.

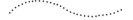

I wasn't exactly new to the two-week wait. A few times before, Dan and I had had not-very-careful sex when we weren't trying for a baby. We knew that forgoing protection would open the door to some outsized possibilities, and we took the risk anyway.

Although I didn't feel ready for a baby yet, I secretly loved the idea of being pregnant, and I especially loved the idea of it happening by almost-accident, like serendipity. There was something about an accidental pregnancy that felt safe because it would mean skipping the uncertainty of trying, the pain of waiting, and the fear that pregnancy might never happen.

It was during that first two-week wait that I became familiar with the term *two-week wait*—the painfully long stretch between ovulation and the first day of your expected period. I finally understood why it's such a selling point that some pregnancy tests can give accurate readings up to five days before a missed period.

My discovery of this term started out innocently enough: I Googled "Are sore breasts a sign of pregnancy?" With that single action, I fell down the internet rabbit hole of trying-to-conceive discussion boards. In those two weeks, I searched every possible symptom and twinge, and what I found was that nearly everything that could be a sign of a normal period on its way—cramping, sore breasts, and irritability, just to name a few—could also be a sign of pregnancy. It's a cruel cosmic joke that keeps us women waiting and guessing and predicting and hoping until the very last minute, when either the test is positive or the first smear of blood shows up on toilet paper.

Up to this point, each of my two-week waits had ended with the latter—along with a few negative tests buried in the garbage.

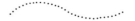

Years later, when I began to think about maybe, possibly, someday trying for a second baby, one of the things I dreaded most was enduring the two-week wait. If you've ever waited for something good—for Christmas to come, for a vacation to roll around, or for a friend to arrive from out of town—you know the delight of the anticipation and how maddeningly fun it is to count the days as they tick closer and closer to the event. And if you've ever waited for something less than pleasant—for pain to relent, for a much-needed surgery, or for an answer or a diagnosis—you know the anxiety that consumes you and how agonizing it is to count down those same days. The two-week wait feels like both kinds of waiting at once, but you don't know which ending will be yours: the joy or the grief.

When I've asked my friends about their experiences with the two-week wait, many of them admitted to spending an embarrassing amount of time on discussion boards, overanalyzing and over-Googling every little cramp. When I first started reading these discussions, I thought it was all in good fun—a rite of passage, even. It was a way to keep hope alive, to cheer on other women who hoped their waiting would end with two pink lines.

There is power in reading other people's stories, in catching a spark of their hope and fanning it into flame for ourselves. I wasn't ready to tell anyone but my closest friend that I was trying for a baby, so it was a gift to have thousands of other women's stories at my fingertips and to realize I wasn't the only one feeling anxious, overanalyzing every symptom, and struggling to get through the two-week wait.

But over time, my reading became maniacal. Instead of adding to my reserves of hope, reading these discussion boards began to deplete me. The more I read, the hungrier I became for one more minute, one more story, one more click—and I started to feel frantic and coiled inside, like a tightly wound spring.

It was nearly impossible to focus on anything else when the discussion boards were calling to me. I remember sitting on my couch one Friday night, a hot cup of tea in hand, ready to finish Jane Austen's *Persuasion*. It was an introvert's dream—Dan was out late at a work event, it had been a long week at work for me, and I had the apartment all to myself on a chilly winter evening. After posting a picture of my setup on Instagram, I opened my browser to look up *this one teeny-tiny thing*, and when I surfaced an hour later, I noticed my tea had gone cold and I was too tired to find out whether Captain Wentworth and Anne Elliot would finally confess their feelings to each other. I had wasted my whole evening feeling frantic and trying to satisfy my inner hunger rather than caring for myself in a refreshing, meaningful way.

Though I'd originally sought hope from these discussion boards, somewhere my search had morphed into a quest for control. If I could find someone with a story exactly like mine who ended up healthily pregnant, I thought, that would mean everything would turn out fine for me too.

It turns out control is a cheap form of hope: control promises that we can be the master of our circumstances, but it slowly, sneakily begins to master *us*, and it does not require an ounce of trust in anyone but ourselves. It zaps us of our ability to be vulnerable with ourselves, with our loved ones, and with God. By taking the full weight of responsibility into our own hands, we mitigate the risk of hoping because we will shoulder all the blame for "failure."

I wish I could tell you I had a profound come-to-Jesus moment in which I realized I just needed to trust God as my real source of hope and learn to be more patient, when I shut my laptop and declared, "No more discussion-board rabbit holes!" While I can't remember a specific moment like that, I do know I was beginning to feel tired and tethered to the wrong thing, and I was beginning to crave real hope over the cheap imitation.

I did get my period that month, and though I felt drawn to the discussion boards to make sense of my disappointment, I instead took my big feelings to my loved ones—people who could speak directly to my sadness because they knew *me*.

So much about pregnancy feels out of our control: whether we can get pregnant, will get pregnant, or will stay pregnant; whether our babies will be healthy; whether we will be good moms. If we let it, the two-week wait can be a practice round for recognizing what is and is not within our power. (Alas, as much as we may want to, we cannot make ourselves be pregnant.) It is a chance to decide, with the first bit of blood announcing a period, how we will respond and what our motivation will be. We can tighten our grip on control and try again. We can give ourselves to despair and give up altogether. Or we can let the current of hope guide us toward what we really want, whether that's to try again or press pause or pursue something new.

Being motivated by hope is not the easy path, especially if you've risked it all every month for years on end. The message we often hear is that all our effort and pain will be worth it in the end. As humans, we desperately want to tie a bow on our difficult experiences. We want to believe that every hardship is worthwhile and will make us better and stronger. While pain has great capacity to teach us, sometimes it's pointless and unfair.

Perhaps what leads us closer to fulfillment is not forging ahead with a single-minded sense of optimism that everything will always be fine, but choosing our next step with a balance of true hope, honest desire, and hard-won resilience.

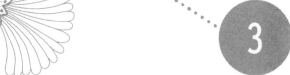

3

Two Pink Lines

I tried my best to ignore the maybe-pregnancy-but-probably-period symptoms during my next cycle. For the most part, I managed to restrain myself from reading discussion boards, but the more difficult task was trying to ignore what my own body was saying. My breasts were uncharacteristically sore, I was experiencing intense emotional swings, and I found myself crying even more than usual. I'm admittedly a crier, but breaking down in tears multiple times a day is not my norm.

You've gotten your hopes up before over these very normal period symptoms, I reminded myself. *Don't overthink this.* I sometimes felt anchored by a deep sense of trust that God would provide either a positive test or tender comfort at the end of my two-week wait, but just as often, I tried to suppress hope by being "realistic" and unattached.

I made a promise to myself that this month I wouldn't take a pregnancy test until I was ten days past ovulation. I'd spent too much money in the preceding months on three-packs of the very sensitive, and very expensive, early-response tests. There was one slim stick left, wrapped in pink foil and waiting under my bathroom sink, and I didn't want to pee on five dollars just to get my period later that day.

One night toward the end of my cycle, when I was feeling exceptionally tender and was anticipating blood any day now, I took out my pain on my sister-in-law Ashley. I sat in my warm car in front of my apartment, my phone pressed to my ear, ready to make a run for it through the biting cold as soon as we hung up. My eyes lingered on the snow packed down in the parking lot, gray and sludgy.

Ashley asked gently enough, "How's it going with trying to get pregnant?"

Before I could exert any restraint, tears burned at the back of my eyes and began to spill onto my cheeks, my breath became ragged, and my heart raced. Ashley and I were already in a tough spot—we'd had an argument a few days before and were trying to work it out—and her question, though she had asked it because she genuinely cared, felt like an imposition, an invasion, a reminder of what I wanted but did not have.

My reaction was unfair; she didn't mean it that way, and I knew it. But, pregnant or not, I turn into the worst version of myself when my hormones run wild at the end of my cycle. It always feels a bit like the people who love me most have decided to rub me raw just to see how much it will take for me to snap. And this time, I did.

I could tell my period was coming the next day, and as much as I'd tried to remind myself that *it will be okay, this wasn't my month, I'll have another chance*, the disappointment had found a way in, worming itself into my heart and beginning its metamorphosis into bitterness.

An achy lump filled my throat and I choked out a tense "I'm not ready to talk about this," then mumbled that I had to go and I'd call her back another day.

I stepped out of the car, the frigid air freezing the tears to my face. I pulled my hood over my head and retreated back inside myself as I dashed through the cold.

I woke up the next morning, ten days past ovulation, at 4:30. I rolled onto my stomach and noticed that for the first time in a week I could lie on my chest without pain. With the disappearance of that tenderness, the last tiny glimmer of hope—which I had tried to pretend was not there—began to disappear too, like the last embers of a fire fading from orange to black.

I grabbed the basal thermometer from my bedside table, popped it into my mouth, and closed my eyes as I listened to the *beep . . . beep . . . beep* that had become the opening song of my daily soundtrack. I was expecting to see the standard temperature drop, indicating my period was on its way, but I was surprised to find my temperature was still high. It had spiked, in fact.

Maybe?

Not wanting to wake up Dan, I tiptoed to the guest bathroom, flipped on the too-bright lights, and sat down on the toilet. I let out a bit of the precious first-thing-in-the-morning urine—the stuff the test instructions tell you to use—and discovered no blood. I wasn't sure how to feel about this. That tiny bit of hope began to flicker again—first as a spark in my stomach, sending fire toward my chest—but I also felt tempted to put it out myself, preemptively protecting my heart from being burned. But what I felt most strongly was insatiable curiosity.

I grabbed my last early-response test from under the sink, along with a disposable plastic cup. *Am I really going to do this? Am I really going to use my last test?* I tried to convince myself to wait until tomorrow, but curiosity drove me forward.

I peed into the little white cup, tore through the pink foil wrapping of the test, and dipped the stick. I watched my urine seep through the tiny window as I had so many times before. The control line appeared immediately—bright and pink and utterly alone. Negative.

I tossed the test aside and scrubbed my hands a bit too hard, chiding myself for getting my hopes up at the last second, feeling silly and wasteful and naïve. I picked up the test to toss it in the trash, and there it was: a faint but visible second pink line.

No, this can't possibly be right, I told myself. But I knew I was well within the ten-minute window of the test's reliability. I closed my eyes and looked again, trying to dislodge the image in case it was a shadow or my imagination. When I opened my eyes again, cautiously, tentatively, the line was still there. I put the test down, the plastic clicking against the countertop, and then I picked it up again. The line was *still* there.

I studied myself in the mirror and noticed my bedhead, the powder-blue shorts I slept in every night, the totally unassuming and unchanged way I looked, despite the seismic shift that had just occurred. A small smile formed on my lips, and I tried to suppress it, still not fully believing the results.

It was supposed to be hard for me to get pregnant, I thought. *It was supposed to take months, a year, two years.* I smiled again and this time let it linger for a moment. *What if this is real?*

I grabbed a dollar-store test, thinking this one would surely be negative. Dollar-store tests are wonderfully cheap but not super sensitive, so I figured a positive on this test would prove it to me. Five minutes later, I saw a bright, bold control line and the faintest-of-faint results line—this one was positive too. A tiny giggle bubbled up from my throat, coupled with a gasp for air.

I'm not typically one for whole-body expressions of my spirituality: at church, my arms stay firmly at my sides, though occasionally I'll sway if I think no one is watching me. But in that moment, all I could do was drop to my knees and press my face into the cold tile floor of our guest bathroom, gently rocking back and forth. I whispered over and over, "Thank you, thank you, thank you, thank you." And when I could form more words, "Please make it stick. Please keep us strong."

When I eventually moved on with my regular morning routine, I couldn't stop smiling and thinking about the teeny-tiny life growing inside me that very minute. Settling into my usual spot on our brown couch—the first big purchase Dan and I made after getting married— I pulled my favorite fuzzy blanket around my soon-to-be-growing body and opened my phone to read a Lenten devotional email.

This particular message was written by a woman who had recently learned she was pregnant—a wild coincidence considering what had happened to me moments before. The shared experience sparkled inside me for a moment and then fizzled out as I read that it was her fourth pregnancy, but so far, only one of her previous three babies had survived. She wrote of her disbelief and joy at this positive pregnancy test, emotions that were quickly overtaken by fear: "Dear God, don't let my baby die." I felt the breath rush out of me as I started to cry—for the joy of new life, for the sorrow of lost babies, and as a way of opening the release valve to let off some of the overwhelm and disbelief I was feeling.

I began to write out a prayer asking God for safety, protection, and provision for me, for this stranger writing to me from across the internet, and for the precious babies who were making their homes in our wombs. I prayed for my friends who were facing infertility, who were longing for children, who had yet to see their two pink lines. Joy and sorrow and guilt and longing swirled together in my chest as I tried to make sense of this gift.

It can be disorienting when we finally receive something we've been longing for, whether it's a pregnancy or a relationship or an award or an achievement. We can struggle to accept the gift for ourselves when it feels unfair—why us and not our just-as-deserving friend? But good gifts are not a zero-sum game; receiving something we've desired doesn't lessen the chances of someone else receiving their wished-for outcome too. We don't need to reject the gift or try to minimize it in our own hearts. Perhaps the best we can do is to accept it gratefully and pray that it will be a quiet source of hope (rather than a source of hurt) for someone who needs a dose of belief and possibility. We can pray that we'll get the chance to share in a loved one's joy when their long-awaited dream is finally fulfilled.

I could hardly believe what was happening. Everything had changed, and yet everything felt the same—I certainly didn't feel pregnant. But on that cold March morning, when the world felt gray and icy and dead, I dared to hope that maybe spring was coming, that maybe new life was emerging. I let myself revel in the warmth and weight of pure joy.

To Tell or Not to Tell

4

While Dan and I were trying for a baby, I thought of a million fun ways to tell him when I finally got pregnant. Maybe I'd wrap the pregnancy test in baby-shower wrapping paper or leave a onesie lying around the apartment. I could present him with a book about fatherhood or find a casual but clever way to work it into a conversation.

But when I saw those two pink lines, the ones I thought wouldn't be coming for me this month, I didn't want to wait to create the perfect moment. I needed to tell him the news that was not just mine but *ours*. I needed him to share in my joy and fear. It felt like the world was shifting around me, and I hoped the act of telling him about this growing poppy seed would ground me in what was real.

I decided if Dan was awake before I left for work, I'd tell him right away, but if he wasn't, I wouldn't wake him up intentionally. I wanted him to be fully conscious for that kind of news. While I was cooking my breakfast, Dan stumbled out of our bedroom. He was obviously tired but possibly coherent enough for a life-changing conversation. I tested him with a few low-level questions: "How did you sleep?" and then "Do you have any work appointments tonight?" It was an unsuspicious question— Dan is a real estate agent, so he often works evenings.

He told me he'd be showing a house at six thirty and wouldn't be home until close to eight o'clock. I thought I might lose my mind if I had to wait that long to tell him, so I decided to go for it, right there in the tiny kitchen of our first apartment. My thoughts raced in that small downbeat of the conversation as I debated what my delivery should be: *Should I say it with a big smile? An excited shout? A nonchalant tone? Should I look him in the eye or casually let it slip as I flip my chicken sausage?* I was about to speak the words that would change our world—and the power was a little intimidating.

I looked up from the sweet potatoes that were sizzling on the stove, and I began to mumble, gaining confidence and excitement as I went: "Well, I thought about waiting to tell you in some cute way . . . but I can't wait until eight tonight. I'm pregnant!"

A brief smile flickered across his face as he looked at me through his still-sleepy eyes, trying to process what I'd said.

"You're pregnant?" He let out a short laugh and then asked, "Are you serious? Are you really?"

Before I could turn off the stove, he'd wrapped me in one his bear hugs, and I breathed him in—the smell of his skin first thing in the morning, the feel of his stubble against my cheek. His solidity grounded me in this moment, just as I had hoped it would.

We lingered in the kitchen for a few more minutes, talking and dreaming. By now, I was running very late for work, but I didn't want to leave the protective bubble of this moment, bursting it as I closed our apartment door. I wanted to stay right there with Dan, where I didn't have to face my fears about what might happen, where this pregnancy felt real and safe and ordained.

Besides, how could I possibly go to work? How could I focus on anything else when this mind-blowing process was unfolding in my body? When everything had changed?

Once I had pushed the limit of how late I could be, I kissed Dan goodbye and left for the office with a second person in tow.

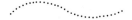

The next person I told about my pregnancy was the receptionist at my OB-GYN's office. I called her from my car after arriving at work, knowing there'd be no privacy at my cubicle. After verifying my personal information and asking my reason for requesting an appointment ("Um, a home pregnancy test was faintly positive, so I think I'm pregnant?"), she asked, "Which hospital will you be delivering at?"

What? Her question caught me off guard. *I had a positive home pregnancy test and now I'm making delivery plans?*

I sputtered, "West Fulton, I think."

"When was the first day of your last menstrual period?"

"February 9."

"Okay . . ." She trailed off for a moment before announcing, "That means your due date is November 16! Congratulations!"

My . . . due date?

The reality of this pregnancy hit me all over again. This wasn't just an abstract dream for the future. It wasn't just a positive test or faint pink line. It was a life, a baby, a real little person that would be born to us in November.

After I hung up the phone, I put a shaky, sweaty hand up to my face and shook my head softly. Gratitude surged in my heart for this tiny new creation. But I still felt deep sorrow and anger for friends who were waiting for their positive tests, anxiety over the possibility of miscarriage, and a staggering realization that I was clueless about all things related to pregnancy. It was as if the blood leaving my heart was oxygenated with happiness but returned through my veins depleted of its vitality, lacking life and goodness.

Rising to the surface, though, the way heat rises through a house on a chilly day, was unspeakable, radiant joy. I let the waves of emotion carry me for a few minutes, right there in my car as winter continued to swirl around me. The world didn't look all that different from last night, when I'd sat in a parking lot talking to my sister-in-law—slushy snow, gray skies, a bite in the air—but the invisible shift inside me was palpable. What filled me now was hope.

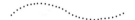

I carried my sweet secret around with me for the rest of the day, and my whole body lit up every time I remembered my poppy-seed baby. I was hungry for information that would help me make sense of what was happening, so I downloaded a few pregnancy apps and read about what my body was already doing at four weeks along. But most of all, I was bursting to tell someone, anyone, my news—eager to experience the rush of reality that came with speaking it aloud.

Later that night, Dan and I discussed who we would tell and when. I talked to my mom almost every day on my way home from work, so I knew I wouldn't be able to keep the secret from her for long. We made plans to tell her first and in person, and to tell his parents as soon as possible too.

As excited as I was to tell people, I was also starting to feel nervous. For me, fear tends to creep in after the sun goes down, and it was true that night: as darkness fell outside, darkness began to take root in my mind. I wondered whether it was silly to share the news so early, before we reached the "safety" of the second trimester—and in some twisted way, I thought telling people might bring bad luck. I get a little superstitious about following the "rules," even rules I've made up, so I try to do and say and think all the right things to avoid inviting heartache. If I assumed this pregnancy would go smoothly, would that lead to complications? If I believed everything would be fine, would I miscarry? If I expected the worst, could that guarantee the best?

Like a balloon with a slow leak, I began to deflate from the excited mom-to-be I had been that morning. I tried to push away the hope that had buoyed me a few short hours ago. Miscarriage is common in the early weeks of pregnancy, and I didn't want to look foolish for counting on something that didn't yet belong to me, for taking possession of a gift I might have to give back.

Keeping this pregnancy between me and Dan (and my OB-GYN) seemed like a way to protect myself against potential pain. If I didn't let myself get attached to this baby, then maybe dealing with grief wouldn't be so hard. And in some strange way, I thought if I let people get excited for me, I would disappoint them if I miscarried. Maybe it would be better to forgo vulnerability now, I thought, in order to spare everyone pain in the future.

But pain and vulnerability don't work that way.

I prayed honestly about my fears over the next few days, my words marked by desperation and superstition. I didn't feel any sort of guarantee from God, nor did I feel the peace I longed for. But I did feel a nudge—toward Dan, toward my family, toward my trusted community of friends. There was no lightning-bolt moment, no audible voice in my ear, but I sensed God leaning toward me and saying, *These are the people I've given to you, and they are the ones who love you like I do. Let them walk you through this.* I began to acknowledge that it might be wise to let some people in—to share with the friends I would want walking beside me and supporting me in whatever came.

Standing shakily on that revelation of wisdom and love, I told my mom I was pregnant. The memory of that moment stands out to me still, as bright and joyful as ever. My mom, my brother, Dan, and I were all standing in her kitchen, breathing in the scent of cooling pizza. Dan and I were house hunting at the time, and I told her I had bought a couple of things for our future home but I would only keep one of the items. I turned around and pulled two sets of newborn pajamas from my bag—a blue-striped pair with tiny bear feet and a cream-colored set with pink roses and ruffles. Realization sparked in her eyes as she shouted, "No! Really? Shush! Are you joking?"

I warned her that I was only five weeks along, and who knew what might happen, and let's not get too excited yet, but she was having none of it. She heard me and understood my fears—she'd had two miscarriages herself—and she assured me she would pray for the baby's health, but she also said she wouldn't hold back on experiencing joy now.

We gradually told more friends and family, and with each announcement, I felt myself softening, unfurling slowly, like the first tulip of spring daring to trust the warmth of the sun and believing that a frost would not come. A growing sense of confidence sprang up within me as beloved friends and family members believed and hoped and trusted on my behalf. Their belief allowed me to slowly believe it for myself— that the miracle was real, that everything might be okay, and that if the worst happened, I wouldn't have to grieve alone.

My friend Stephanie says it perfectly: "We're not meant to do faith alone; we need each other. When we get weary, we need someone else's hope to cover the gap for us. . . . [W]e need each other along the way— in the celebrations, when the answer is yes; in the heartbreaks, when the answer is no; and in the agonizing middle, when the answer is wait."[2]

We can't prevent heartbreak, and we can't guarantee good fortune. But we can invite other people to walk the road with us when it

---

2 Stephanie Rische, "Don't Do Belief Alone," *Stephanie Rische* (blog), January 17, 2018, http://www.stephanierische.com/dont-do-belief-alone.

appears treacherous and unknown. The connection born out of vulnerability—with God, with ourselves, with our loved ones—doesn't make the journey safer, but it certainly makes it richer.

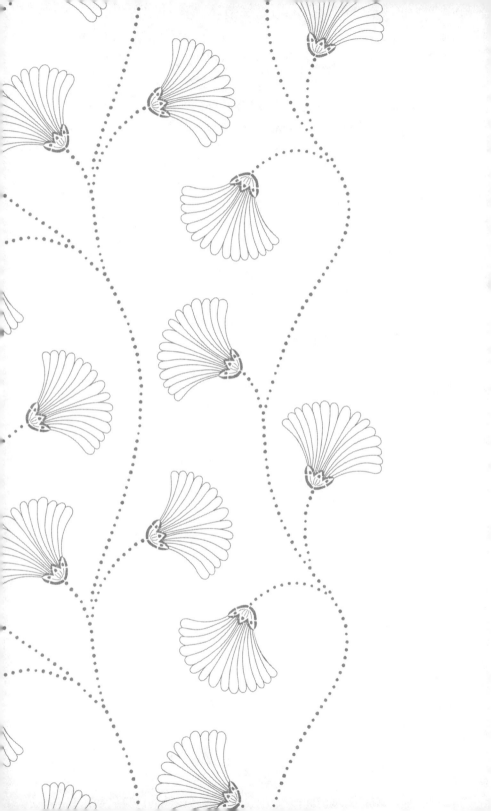

5

Fed Is Best

I started gagging before the fork even reached my mouth.

It was a normal Monday about seven weeks into my pregnancy, and I had brought my normal lunch to work: leftover grilled chicken and roasted broccoli. When 12:30 rolled around, I popped my lunch container into the office microwave, brought it back to my desk, and felt my stomach lurch.

Has this broccoli gone bad? Why does it smell so putrid? I wondered. *Was the chicken this rubbery last night? Why didn't Dan tell me? How could anyone eat this?*

The heaving that followed was a rite of passage: the onset of morning sickness, even at lunchtime.

I choked down a few bites as I distracted myself by scrolling Instagram, and eventually I gave up and put more than half of my lunch back in the fridge.

It's not exactly pleasant to be ready to retch at any given moment and to constantly wonder whether you're within sprinting distance of a bathroom, just in case. But in addition to the nausea, something else was bubbling up from my churning stomach: relief, and a strange sense of excitement.

Morning sickness is perhaps the most classic pregnancy symptom. We've all seen movies depicting women who don't know they're pregnant until they're hugging a toilet and counting backward to figure out when their last period was. Nausea is an initiation of sorts, a physical manifestation of the fact that our worlds are being turned upside down, leaving us more than a little woozy. For me, the sickness was a welcome reminder of the extreme changes happening in my body and a reassurance that everything was progressing as it was supposed to. The baby was eating up all my energy and blood sugar, and my hormones were exploding.

Over the next few weeks, I noticed my nausea followed a predictable pattern. I felt good in the mornings, especially if I nibbled a few pretzels between breakfast and lunch. I could eat about half my lunch before I started to feel sick, but then I was mostly okay the rest of the afternoon. (However, my cubicle was located right across from our department's small kitchen, so every day, I suffered secretly behind my half-walls as people heated up their soup, lasagna, or, most unfortunately for me, fish. I hadn't told many people at work that I was pregnant, and I didn't want to announce it by vomiting at my desk.)

By dinnertime, I couldn't fathom eating anything besides chips, so that's basically what I did. Every few days, I made a big batch of taco meat: ground turkey mixed with ground beef, sautéed with onion and olive oil, and seasoned with some of my favorite spices—cumin, chili powder, garlic. I hid some finely chopped veggies in the mixture, hoping to trick my body into eating them.

Each evening, Dan and I would settle into our oversized armchair with our bowls of meat and a giant bag of tortilla chips between us. I used the chips as a vehicle to get the mixture from the bowl to my stomach—scooping up a tiny amount and chewing quickly, trying not to taste the meat, and focusing instead on the saltiness of the chip. I would start to gag after a few bites and resort to eating just the chips.

Before pregnancy, I had subsisted mostly on meat and produce, avoiding many sources of refined sugar and starches. I indulged in my favorite treats on the weekends—donuts, French toast, takeout from the Chinese place down the street. Looking back, these rules seem arbitrary and unhealthy, but at the time, they gave me a sense of control over my body. I was still recovering from disordered eating, and I hadn't yet learned to make food choices from a place of compassion and desire.

I planned to continue my meat-and-veggie eating habits throughout pregnancy, partly because I genuinely wanted to put "healthy" foods into the body I was sharing with my baby and partly because I was terrified of gaining weight. It's normal and good and necessary to gain weight while pregnant, but it also triggered many old but not-quite-buried feelings.

It was a powerful shift that when faced with the choice between eating nothing and eating pretzels, between gagging on chicken or gobbling kettle-cooked chips, I chose the latter—even though they were foods I had deemed "bad." These moments were my first lesson in "fed is best," a catchphrase we hear in mommy circles that celebrates all the ways moms feed their babies: breastmilk, formula, purées, table food, puffs, rice cereal, and everything in between. It turns out fed is best for babies in utero, too, as well as for the moms who carry them.

Eating something was obviously better than eating nothing, but even so, I faced a real sense of failure. I was ashamed at how much weight I was putting on. I was embarrassed at how quickly I'd reneged on my intentions. I felt frustrated that I couldn't do what I considered to be the "best" thing for my child or for myself. This was also, necessarily, my first lesson in self-compassion. My instinct was to beat myself up over every bite of less-than-ideal food, but eventually I grew tired of doing that all day, every day. Carbs were a temporary cure for the nausea, and so I ate them—hesitantly at first, and eventually with abandon. And in doing so, they became a gateway to deeper healing in my relationships with food and with my body.

Everyone will tell you their tricks for curbing the sickness: consuming Preggie Pops, eating a single saltine before getting out of bed, or drinking a glass of water upside down whenever the nausea creeps in. Some people might tell you it will pass if you just hang on, or they might tell you their own horror stories of puking in the middle of giving a presentation, or they might tell you to be happy you're having a baby at all.

I want you to imagine me holding your shoulders (or holding your hair back), looking you in the eye, and telling you the truth: It's okay to hate this part. It's okay to strangely enjoy this part. It's okay to take a nap every day during the time when you're most nauseated. It's okay to wonder how on earth you'd survive another pregnancy and to think you might be cut out to do this only once. It's okay to accept or *ask* for help when you don't know how you'll survive another trip to the grocery store, surrounded by all that food and all those smells and all those people who don't understand the concept of personal space. It's okay to wish this time away. It's okay to secretly seethe when someone says, "I never got sick with any of my pregnancies!" or when someone else tries to one-up your experience with their more extreme story. It's okay to resent your body and wonder whether this is even worth it.

None of this means you're not grateful to be pregnant. It means you're a human who's growing an actual parasite (even if it's a sweet and desired parasite) that is causing your body to do things such as alter your hormonal makeup and crave chicken nuggets at midnight and vomit those nuggets twenty minutes later.

Our culture places enormous and often unfair pressure on women to push through difficult times, keep the plates spinning, and not show anyone we don't have it all under control. We're not allowed to give the impression that we are anything less than capable, and so we understandably struggle to face our limitations, much less let anyone else see them. Basically, we're expected to be superheroes.

Along the same line, there's an oft-repeated joke about the difference between a man-cold and a woman-cold: The woman continues juggling her kids, her job, her house, and everything else. The man, by contrast, is laid up in bed, acting as if he is really and truly about to die. I get a deep sense of validation from this, because even though I love my husband dearly, he very much falls into the man-cold stereotype. It's easy for us to roll our collective eyes at these "fragile" men . . . but I wonder whether we could use this stereotype to push back on some of the pressure we feel to be all things and do all things well at all times.

Our responsibilities are real and important, and we can't always put our lives on hold simply because we feel a bit under the weather. But if our can-do attitudes have led us to a different and possibly more damaging extreme of never taking a break, putting too much stock in our own abilities, or forcing ourselves to keep calm and carry on, then what we should really do is ask for help, crawl into bed and rest, and celebrate ourselves for doing so.

Pregnancy nausea can likewise force us to face our limitations, beckon us to be gentle with ourselves, and invite us to nourish our bodies in unexpected ways. And sometimes the best way to do all three is to eat tortilla chips for dinner . . . again.

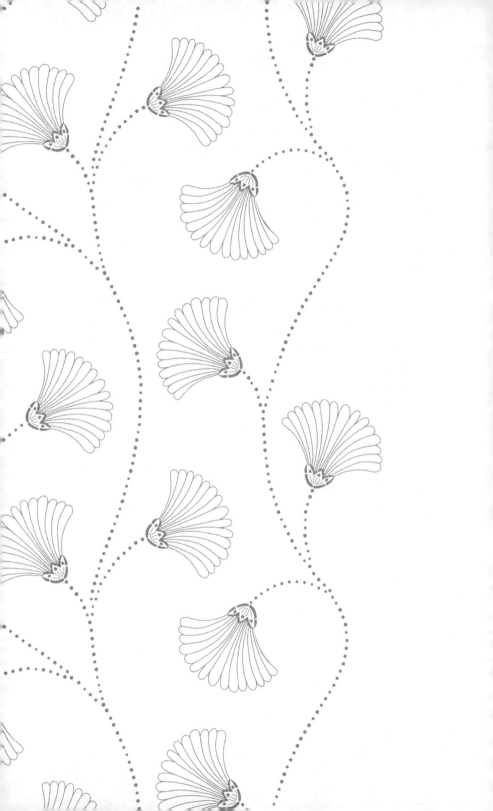

6

Miscarriage Scare

Is that blood? I was standing in a crowded bookstore when I felt a strange dampness, and my mind started to race. Almost immediately, I jumped to an extreme conclusion: *I must be having a miscarriage.* I was suddenly desperate to get to a bathroom so I could check what was going on.

It's astonishing, really, how quickly my mind can lead me to worst-case scenarios, even with no evidence to back up my fears.

I had met up with some of my work friends at a book launch for one of our favorite authors. We were standing at the back of the room near the doors, which had been left open to allow an uncharacteristically warm March breeze to blow through, ruffling our hair and reminding us that winter was finally, mercifully ending.

The author had just started her talk, and my heart pounded wildly as I scanned for a restroom sign. My eyes landed on one at the far end of the store, but there were too many people packed in front of me. I couldn't move. I have no memory what the author talked about that day because my mind was stuck in a cruel, intrusive loop: *I'm losing the baby, I'm losing the baby, I'm losing the baby.*

Once the crowd dissipated, I slipped away to the restroom and discovered everything was fine; I'd been feeling normal discharge. Relief replaced panic in the pit of my stomach, and I felt safe again . . . at least until the next time my mind got the better of me.

I wish there were a nicer way to say this—that I struggled with fear, or that I worried a little more than I should have. But the truth is, I was completely consumed by the fear of miscarriage. Imagining worst-case scenarios about this pregnancy took up the majority of my thinking.

The gap between where I was—only a few weeks pregnant—and when I would have my first ultrasound at ten weeks felt like an impassable expanse of time. *What if I get to the appointment and find out the "baby" is nothing more than an empty sac? What if the technician discovers the pregnancy is ectopic? Will I see a bean-sized baby on the screen but be told the words every mother dreads: "I'm sorry, but there's no heartbeat"? How can I possibly wait until ten weeks to know whether this baby is alive? What if I'm growing attached just to be wrenched apart from my already-beloved child?* My emotions felt like taut wires, ready to snap. If I lost this baby, I feared I would be sliced in half, and my heart and my faith might never recover.

I tried to remind myself that God was in control, but that idea didn't provide comfort. At best, it felt like an empty platitude, and at worst, it felt cruel: if God was in control and I miscarried, what would that mean? I knew plenty of people of faith who had experienced pregnancy loss. Why would praying make any difference for me and for this child?

Every time I started to feel hopeful and believe this pregnancy might last, I would hear a story of miscarriage at eight weeks, eleven weeks, fifteen weeks, and I would grow terrified again. I was afraid that the very act of hoping would cause my hopes to be dashed; that the moment I started to dream, my dreams would be crushed. I could already hear the well-meaning voices of family and friends and church ladies: *God had a plan, and you can always try again.* But I didn't want to try again for another child in a few months; I wanted *this* one, *this* child, *this* gift.

With every little twinge of pain, I imagined the pregnancy was ectopic and called my doctor just to be sure. Every time I went to the bathroom, I feared I would find blood. I religiously checked the toilet paper each time I wiped, making sure it was clean and clear.

I made it through the days one bathroom trip at a time and marked the days one by one in my head, breathing a sigh of relief each morning when I woke up still pregnant. I tallied the weeks the way I tally my writing word counts or weekly work hours: moving ahead slowly, one step at a time.

But on Easter Sunday, when I was eight weeks pregnant, I woke up, went to the bathroom, and found what I'd been fearing from the moment I took the pregnancy test: blood. Not pinkish spotting like I've heard is normal, but fresh, sticky, purple-red bits of tissue. It wasn't a lot—not even enough to make it into the toilet—but it was there on the paper, the crimson smear a stark contrast against the sanitary white.

My body responded before my mind did: my limbs went cold, like all the blood had rushed out through my toes, and my heart began to race. After all those weeks of worrying and then feeling peace, growing anxious and then finding rest and reassurance, it seemed clear that this pregnancy was ending.

I walked back to my bedroom on shaky legs and placed a hand on Dan's shoulder to wake him up. He'd barely opened his eyes before I told him what was happening and that everything was not okay. He lay there quietly, his reaction impossible to read.

I pressed him for a response, unsure whether I wanted to hear his usual optimism or have him sit in the grief with me. He finally said, in his cool and measured manner, "Well, I feel sad that this is happening, and awful about how worried you are. But I don't feel concerned. I think everything is fine."

Even though his words should have been reassuring, my telling someone else what was happening made it feel even more real. In the same way that telling Dan about the positive test had grounded me in the reality of the pregnancy, telling him about the blood grounded me in the possibility of losing it. The tears I'd been too shocked to shed at first burst forth now. I sank onto the bed, sobbing and gasping for air.

The thought of getting dressed and going to church felt daunting, and making it through the whole Easter service, impossible. I wouldn't be able to think about anything but the health of the baby. I certainly wouldn't get through those ninety minutes without crying, and since I hadn't told many people at church, I didn't want to have to explain myself. But I also knew that staying home—wallowing and worrying, running to the bathroom every few minutes to check for stains on the toilet paper, waiting around for cramping to start—would drive me mad. So we went.

The tone of the service was victorious and certain, celebrating the triumph of life over death. I tried to sing along with the worship team, but every time I managed to squeak out a few words, my lips and shoulders would start to quiver, and fresh, hot tears would flow down my cheeks. Eventually I stopped trying to participate vocally and instead closed my eyes, letting everyone else's words wash over me. I imagined the people around me singing on my behalf and expressing the certainty I wanted to believe but couldn't: *Because he lives, I can face tomorrow. Because he lives, every fear is gone. I know he holds my life (my baby's life), my future (my baby's future) in his hands.*[3]

In my mind, I begged God to resurrect this pregnancy, but I couldn't help dwelling on what it would mean about God's character if I miscarried. If God had the power to make this all okay but chose not to, was God still good? And who was I to bother God with this request when there is so much large-scale suffering in the world? With all the ways I experience privilege, why should God spare me any pain?

Dan and I had been planning to tell the last of our family members about the pregnancy later that day: my little sister, Maddie, in person at

---

3 Matt Maher, artist, "Because He Lives (Amen)," by Chris Tomlin, Daniel Carson, Ed Cash, et al., track 13 on *Saints and Sinners*, Provident, 2015.

Easter dinner; Dan's brother and sister-in-law over the phone later that night. The bleeding hadn't stopped by the time we arrived at my mom's house, and I questioned whether it was worth telling Maddie. Could I bear her excitement knowing it might all be ending this very moment, that the baby might already be dead? Dan still believed I wasn't miscarrying, as did my friend Eileen, a nurse I'd texted earlier in my panic.

"As long as you don't start cramping and soaking pads, there's no reason to believe you're miscarrying," her text reassured me. "Spotting and bleeding—even bright red blood—can be very normal during the first trimester as your uterus is stretching rapidly. Sometimes a little blood escapes, and it's no big deal. You'll have to wait and see, but I would guess it's normal."

Her professional opinion was a comfort, and Dan encouraged me to believe her and to tell our family members about the pregnancy anyway. His gentle insistence that we share the news, even as I was unsure what the next day or the next hour would hold, reminded me of God's nudge from a few weeks before: *Let people in. Let me love you through them.*

I felt God's nearness in their mixture of excitement and empathy, which carried me through the rest of the day. I felt it in the permission they gave me to be upset and in their unabashed desire to celebrate the life I was growing today. Speaking the news out loud despite my doubts, and letting other people believe and celebrate on my behalf, helped me see this pregnancy as a gift—even if the day's events felt like anything but.

Pregnancy is not a gift God hangs over our heads, reminding us to be grateful for it or else. God does not sadistically string us along with the intention of breaking our hearts. Even with all the chaos and pain and suffering that's present in our world, we are allowed to worry about these tiny lives and to be heartsick over the thought of losing them— they are a part of us, one with us, created within our very own bodies. God doesn't desire for us to be anxious, but it's understandable that we would feel distress or that we'd worry about all the things that might go wrong. It shows that our hearts are already developing the instincts of a mother. God is there with us in every anxious thought, ready to comfort us moment by moment, ready to mourn or celebrate with us in whatever comes.

Pregnancy is a gift meant to be *enjoyed* for however long we have it. We carried life, whether it was for two weeks or forty-two.

And if each day with our babies is a gift, then even if today is the last one, it is both something to grieve and something to treasure.

7

First Ultrasound

Dan and I sat in standard-issue hospital waiting-room chairs and listened for my name to be called. I crossed and uncrossed my legs, uncomfortable from all the water I'd had to drink in preparation for the ultrasound. My foot bobbed up and down, and I studied the carpet underneath my shoes: muted green and blue swirls. I generally hate hospitals, but I took comfort in how familiar this one felt, even though I'd never been there before. The neutral paint on the walls, the generic chairs, and the design of the carpet all lent a sense of predictability to a moment that felt unstable.

As soon as the phone lines had opened on Monday morning, I'd called my doctor to report that I was bleeding and to see whether I should come in. After a painstaking couple of hours, a nurse called me back, and I dashed from the not-so-privacy of my cubicle to a nearby conference room to take the call.

She asked me to tell her the whole story, and when I finished, she asked how I was doing now. I told her the bleeding had mostly stopped, but there were some bits of blood every now and then. She reiterated exactly what my nurse friend had told me the day before: since there was no cramping and the flow never got heavier, everything was probably fine, and a little bit of bleeding is normal and common during the first trimester.

"At this point, the baby is too small for us to hear the heartbeat with a doppler in the office," she told me. "But if you're feeling worried, I can try to get you in for an ultrasound this week. Are you open to other locations besides your regular office?"

I would have driven to Canada if it meant confirming the health and safety of this baby. "Yes," I said. "Definitely open to other locations."

She scheduled me for an appointment that evening at a hospital about thirty minutes from my apartment. And so I continued waiting and checking, waiting and checking—praying each time that I wouldn't suddenly find more blood, reminding myself each time to find joy in the present.

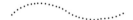

Dan had met me in the parking lot of the hospital after work that night. He tried to distract me from my nervousness by talking about what it would be like to arrive at our hospital later that year—me walking in pregnant and then being wheeled out with a baby in my arms.

I smiled tightly at his attempt. As much as I appreciated what he was trying to do, my mind was stuck on the possibilities that lay on the other side of those hospital doors. I was feeling more hopeful than I had the day before, as I played the nurse's words over and over in my mind: *This is probably normal; it doesn't sound like a miscarriage.* But it was hard not to imagine the ultrasound technician speaking those other, dreaded words: *I'm sorry, but there's no heartbeat.*

The technician finally emerged from behind the door and called my name, then led us through a series of hallways to the darkened ultrasound room. She explained that she would try to do the scan abdominally first.

"Is your bladder full?" she asked.

"Very full," I confirmed.

"I'm going to try to find the baby and take my pictures. Then I'll turn the screen around and show you what I saw."

She squirted cold gel on my belly and pressed the transducer firmly into my skin, making me squirm and wiggle with the need to pee. She stood straight-faced in front of her screen, giving nothing away as she moved the wand around.

"You seem to be measuring small for how many weeks you are, so I can't see much this way. I'll give you a few minutes to use the bathroom, and then we'll try transvaginally."

I leapt at the chance to use the bathroom, but the relief that came from emptying my bladder was matched by my dismay: *I'm measuring small? How small? Is that normal, or does it mean there's probably no baby in there?* The root of all these questions—perhaps the root of every anxious thought I'd had in the first trimester—was this: *Can I trust my body to do what it's supposed to do? Will it grow and sustain life?*

When I came back from the bathroom, I climbed back onto the exam table and covered myself with the thin hospital blanket. Just as I opened my mouth to ask Dan for reassurance, the technician knocked on the door.

She explained how the internal exam would work: it wouldn't hurt, but I would feel the pressure of the wand against my cervix, and it might dislodge a little more blood over the next few days. As soon as she inserted the wand, I heard a rush of noise, a steady *whoosh-whoosh-whoosh* filling the room. My heart soared, as I assumed this was the baby's heartbeat, but almost as if she could hear my thoughts, the technician said, "That's the sound of your blood moving through the uterus." Well then.

I felt the wand twisting as she checked my ovaries and tubes, heard the *click, click, beep* as she captured image after image. I stared straight up and counted ceiling tiles, then counted the lines on a medical beaker sitting on the counter across from me. I willed her to go faster, willed time to move along, willed my baby to be alive and well. As before, the technician's face told me nothing: she focused only on her screen and carefully completed her work. Every now and then I would look up at Dan, and he'd put his hand on my shoulder and give it a squeeze.

The procedure couldn't have lasted more than fifteen minutes, but in those minutes it felt as though everything I'd hoped for and experienced over the last few months hung in the balance. I was either pregnant or not. My baby was either alive or not. I was either a mother or not. The previous day's revelation settled into my body: whatever happened, I had really been pregnant and really carried life and really been chosen for this particular little one at this moment in time.

I found myself hoping that at the very least, whatever the outcome, the results of the ultrasound would simply be *clear*. I didn't want to hear a vague explanation that it was too early to know whether the baby was okay and be asked to come back next week to have another look. Living in limbo is my version of hell, and if I was going to receive bad news, I wanted the delivery to be direct and swift. As I waited for the words that would change everything, I was strangely at peace for the first time—not certain everything would be okay, but certain *I* would be okay someday.

Finally, the technician turned the screen to face us and pointed out a tiny jelly-bean-shaped blob. She moved the wand slightly to catch the baby at a different angle, and suddenly four tiny nubs appeared on the little body: arms and legs.

Wonder crackled through my body, starting in my heart and working down to my stomach and then my toes, as I saw the shape of my child for the first time. There weren't any truly defining features yet—the little arm buds and dimpled head didn't exactly look like me or Dan—

but I instantly knew this little person was mine. In spite of the wonder, though, I didn't yet feel relief.

"Is there a heartbeat?" I asked.

She pointed to a white dot flashing on the screen, so small I would have otherwise missed it. "Baby's heart is right there. Do you see that little flicker? It's beating strong and healthy," she confirmed. She wasn't able to offer an explanation for the blood but said everything looked healthy and normal and the doctor would follow up with me.

She printed some pictures for us and made a CD with a few more images, including one she had marked "BABY," with an arrow pointing toward the limbed jelly bean. I floated out of the hospital, staring at the photos and finally believing I'd be holding that same healthy baby in eight months.

The relief I got from the ultrasound seemed complete in the moment, but on my way home, I began to self-sabotage by poking tiny holes in my certainty and joy—though I told myself I was being re-alistic. Once I'd pulled into the parking lot of my apartment complex, I Googled "chances of miscarriage after you've seen the heartbeat at eight weeks."

As Dan and I warmed up our Easter-dinner leftovers, I shared my discoveries with him: "Did you know that once you see the heart beating at eight weeks, the chances of miscarriage drop to only 2 percent? And at ten weeks, the chances are less than 1 percent."

"When exactly did you look all this up?" Dan asked as he lifted a plate out of the microwave.

"Before I came in, while I was sitting in the car. Do you think I should reschedule the ten-week appointment for after we get back from our Seattle trip? If we can't hear the heartbeat before we go, I'd hate to spend the whole trip worrying. Although, I guess I'll worry about the ap-pointment if I postpone it, so maybe I should keep it as it is . . ." I rambled as we carried our plates to the living room.

"Brittany, we just saw our healthy baby an hour ago. You saw the heart beating, and you said yourself the chances of miscarriage at this point are slim. You're still worried?"

"Well, yeah. There's no guarantee."

"Will there ever be?"

His question disrupted my swirling thoughts, allowing me to step outside them and give them a careful, reasoned look.

I had made excuse after excuse for why I was allowed to live in fear during the first trimester. *I have no real means of reassurance. My belly isn't growing, and I can't feel the baby moving yet. I don't even feel pregnant. The risk of miscarriage seems so high, and I could miscarry without bleeding and not know for weeks. There's so much that's unknown, and I don't have a window into my womb so I can see that everything is fine.* But an hour ago, I'd had a window into my womb and seen with my own eyes that the baby was healthy and moving and very much alive, and it *still* wasn't enough. I was exhausted and emotionally whiplashed from worrying, finding some relief, and then falling into the next spiral of anxiety.

It's understandable: my hormones had become temperamental, which left me feeling like a kite on a windy day, being pulled up toward the sky before plummeting back down, over and over again, each rise and fall unpredictable. Everything about pregnancy felt so fragile, as if I could do just one thing wrong and, like a swiftly pulled thread, it would cause the whole tapestry to unravel.

The outcome of this pregnancy was not within my control, but worrying allowed me to believe it was. I kept looking toward the next event—having a normal ultrasound, hearing the heartbeat, hitting week thirteen and making it to the second trimester—thinking surely *that* moment would provide a sense of control, complete certainty, and freedom from fear.

It wouldn't.

Whether you're a mom to the six-week-old embryo inside you, the six-week-old infant in your arms, the six-year-old climbing the steps of the school bus, or the sixteen-year-old taking off in their car for the first time, the role of mother presents constant opportunities to worry, to fear, to imagine nightmares coming to life. If I truly thought the worries would end when I got to the "safe zone" of the second trimester, I had a lot to learn about myself—and about motherhood.

In these first few weeks of my first pregnancy, anxiety had dominated my experience, choking off hope and joy whenever they sprang up. And until the previous day, when I decided to start celebrating this baby for as long as I had him or her in my body, I hadn't tried to choose anything other than my debilitating thoughts. I realize now that I probably should have sought professional help for my anxiety, but I was doing the best I could at the time. I had never fully overcome anxiety in the past—surely I wouldn't stand a chance now, I thought, in this new and overwhelming situation.

Sometimes anxiety and fear are simply not within our control. No matter how much we try to talk ourselves out of the spiraling thoughts, remind ourselves to breathe, or clear our heads by going for a walk, fear can best us. But where before I thought the only options were to give in to fear or to conquer it once and for all, I started to see another possibility: to carry fear with me instead of being carried away by it.

We will have an ever-decreasing amount of control over the health and wellness of our children as they grow, and perhaps it's time to get comfortable sitting with fear without letting it take us over. We may not be able to eliminate our worries, but we don't have to let them steer the ship. We can learn to hold both fear and wonder in the same open hand.

When the doctor called me a few days after the ultrasound, she gave me a fresh chance to practice this tension. She didn't know exactly what had caused the bleeding but said everything looked fine and the baby seemed healthy. I had hoped for a clear explanation, but that wasn't available to me.

Instead, I had a few choices.

I could twist her reassurance into a new reason to worry—if she couldn't find the cause of the bleeding, how could she possibly know everything was okay?

I could swallow my fear, focus only on the fact that the baby was healthy, and try to force myself to feel certain and optimistic.

Or I could let the nonexplanation provoke me to a deep sense of awe: a baby I had been certain was dead was actually alive and thriving in my very own body, taking its sustenance from my blood, its cells dividing and multiplying within me, forming limbs and fingers and toes. When viewed in a different light, the very thing that had caused my fear—my lack of control—could also be seen as a beautiful, bewildering mystery.

This, then, is the mystery of mothering: We lend our bodies to a process we can't see or control or fully comprehend, and we open our wombs and our hearts to another person. In doing so, we open ourselves to new depths of pain and delight.

In this tender space, we are offered a chance to let fear drive us deeper into despair or to let it orient us toward wonder. May we pursue the latter wholeheartedly.

8

Blueberry Baby

"Your baby is the size of a sweet pea!"

"Your baby is the size of a cucumber!"

"Your baby is the size of a pumpkin!"

Every Monday morning, after settling in to my cubicle at work, I would open a pregnancy app on my phone to see what was new with my baby and my body that week.

While I knew my body was changing substantially—hormones skyrocketing, uterus growing, blood volume increasing—those changes were mostly invisible to my eye. My belly wasn't getting rounder yet, and I couldn't feel the baby moving around inside me. I thought about him or her constantly, but much about pregnancy still felt abstract.

Instead, I relied on pregnancy apps and books to tell me what was happening in my womb. These resources often liken babies in utero to various pieces of produce—a sweet pea, a raspberry, a plum. Being new to this growing-a-human thing, I eagerly checked the app every week and devoured the information.

During the early days, I remember being amazed that the heart was beating, the organs were forming, and the eyelids and lips I would someday kiss were developing. After reading about the current week's changes and developments, I would often skip ahead to the next week to satisfy my curiosity and eagerness about what was to come, despite the internal sense that I should to try to savor each week slowly.

At week seven I read that the baby was the size of a blueberry, which was ten thousand times the size he or she had been at conception. The rapid growth was staggering, but even more so was the former smallness—just how small is one ten-thousandth of a blueberry? I let my mind wander, remembering and reinterpreting what my faith told me about my baby's identity as a beloved creation of God: *If I'm a tiny dot on this earth, a mere speck in a universe so expansive that it's beyond my comprehension, then what does that make this blueberry baby? Who is this blueberry baby that God cares for them and is shaping them with God's very own hands?*

As the weeks passed, my blueberry became a lime and then a kumquat and then an avocado. The comparison to fruits and vegetables may seem far-fetched, but I relied on these imperfect descriptors to help me make sense of a truth I could not see for myself. These fruits were concrete, tangible pictures I could ground myself in amid the rapid change and overwhelming nature of the miracle happening inside me. No matter how hard I tried, I couldn't wrap my head around all that my body was doing to grow this baby—but I could picture a peach- or pear-sized being with tiny fingers and toes, the ones I would count and marvel at in a matter of months.

Isn't this what humans do with the divine too? We can't help but wrestle with the idea of something so much greater than us. The Bible is full of metaphors for God: Father, Mother, King, Rock. We take concepts we know and apply them to God to help us understand even a small slice of who God is, to reveal spiritual truths one glimpse at a time.

This is normal human behavior, but there can be a dark side. We like black and white, right and wrong, here and there. We like light over shadow, certainty over doubt, clear explanations over open-ended questions, the knowable over the mysterious. So we make God play by *our* rules, forgetting that God is not boxed in by time or space. We can't fathom a being who operates outside of our limitations, so we fashion a God who reflects our identities, try to squeeze God inside the walls of our churches, attempt to distill God's essence into an arsenal of "right" answers.

All the while, God is waiting for us to open our eyes, to see that God is right in front of us, that God's image is the blueprint for the universe, that God cannot be contained by our bodies or our minds or our theological beliefs. God offers us the sweetness of honey and the nourishment of milk and the substance of bread and the richness of wine, asking us to taste and know that God is good, to touch and know that God is real, to see and know that God is behind it all. God is *in* it all.

Likewise, turning to fact-filled apps and books to try to understand what's happening in our bodies isn't necessarily a bad thing. These resources can equip us with knowledge, which can in turn help us feel more connected to the events unfolding inside us. But what they can't do is fully reveal the beauty and wonder and miracle of a tiny life being created cell by cell inside our bodies, *by* our bodies, following the same pattern that has played out in billions of women across human history. And these books and apps definitely can't assuage all our fears or guarantee everything will turn out fine simply because they contain the "right" answers to our questions.

Early on, I prayed for my growing child nearly every day, ending each prayer with a superstitious petition: *Lord, keep this baby safe. Lord, keep this baby growing. Lord, keep this baby healthy.* I probably wouldn't have admitted it at the time, but deep down I was afraid my prayers had a shelf life. I worried that if I didn't ask God to keep the baby healthy every single time I prayed, my previous prayer would expire, and my child would no longer be safe.

I suppose this was my way of boxing in the divine, of trying to make sense of who God is and how God operates, but meanwhile, I was missing the point. Yes, God is the creator of life and was sustaining my child and causing this mystery to progress inside me. But that doesn't mean God is so fickle as to demand I grovel day in and day out with specific requests or risk losing the life God had placed within me— a life that God loved even more than I did.

I had to accept that no amount of information or compulsive recitations could illuminate the mystery, make the abstract tangible, or give me control over the process.

As I leaned in to the mystery—by letting myself become increasingly astonished at what God had set in motion, at what my body was doing without any intervention from me—I found myself repeating that superstitious prayer less frequently. And as those words tapered off, my grip loosened on who I thought God is. God isn't a puppet master or a manipulator, using pregnancy and my love for this child to increase my fear and, thus, my devotion. This is a God who loves fully, unabashedly, even recklessly; a God who loved my blueberry baby long before I knew about him or her, and who would love this baby for a whole lifetime, however long that turned out to be.

We are critical to the process of pregnancy, of course, but thank goodness we are not fully responsible for every little development. We don't need to say any magic words to make it all work. We get to trust the intricate design of our bodies, which God has empowered and equipped to bear life.

What a gift that we get to grow the next generation inside us.

What a relief that we are not alone in this.

What a wonder that we get to be partners and cocreators with God.

This wasn't a one-and-done lesson for me, and I'm guessing it won't be for you, either. We may continue to learn it over and over through the rest of our pregnancies, through the sleepless nights of new motherhood, and through the meltdowns and mess of raising feisty toddlers.

But the more we are molded into the shape of a mother, the more we can acknowledge this paradox: we have great power but little control. As we acknowledge that, perhaps our prayers can change from desperate pleas to keep our babies safe to wonder-filled affirmations of God's goodness, of God's very essence in it all.

Second Trimester

Facing Uncertainty and Making Space

9

Stability

I handed over a cashier's check for what felt like an absurd amount of money—certainly more than I had ever spent in one sitting. Dan and I had just signed dozens of papers in the cramped conference room of a title company, affirming that yes, we wanted this house, and yes, we would pay back the loan. In exchange, we each received a key to our new home.

The next weekend, with the help of our friends and family, we spent hours crawling along the floors, cleaning the baseboards, taping off the trim, and painting every bit of oak bright white—no small task, especially at fourteen weeks pregnant. Those same devoted loved ones helped us move all our stuff in the next Saturday, and we provided boxes of donuts and pizza and a million thank-yous that didn't seem nearly sufficient. After everyone left, I sank into the cushions of our beloved brown sofa, physically and mentally exhausted but comforted by the unmistakable sensation of being home.

Over the next few weeks I unpacked our dishes, coffee mugs, and pots and pans into the kitchen cabinets. We put our Christmas decorations in the crawl space and our snowboards in the attic. I browsed online for area rugs to warm up (and cover) the mismatched hardwood floors.

One of the primary tensions Dan and I had wrestled with during the house-hunting process was whether we should buy at the top of our budget in hopes that it would be our forever home or buy a lower-priced "starter home" knowing we couldn't predict the needs of our growing family. The wiser thing for us to do was save the money and buy below our budget, but part of me was romanced by the idea of my children growing up in only one place.

As a child, I attended four different elementary schools, one middle school, and two high schools. I've moved more than twenty times and lived in four different states. People often ask whether my dad was in the military. He wasn't, but our moves were tied to him. He was forever chasing something—the next big business opportunity, the next stable job when that big business opportunity fell through— and my family went along for the ride.

I hated all this change as it was happening. My family moved to Georgia the summer before my freshman year of high school, and the whole first week of school, I involuntarily threw up my breakfast every day before the bus came. The mix of nerves and excitement—planning how I might reinvent myself, wondering where I'd sit at lunch, wishing I could be starting high school with my old friends instead of making new ones—was too much for my highly sensitive temperament.

This periodic change also created a strange sort of rhythm in my life. Throughout my childhood, my life was upended every three years or so, and now I find myself expecting—sometimes even craving— regular overhauls.

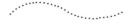

I had been living and teaching in Chicago for two years when I met Dan. Rounding the corner into year three of teaching, I'd made plans to join a close friend the next summer in Spain, where she was already living. We would teach English at a local school and spend our weekends traveling Europe together, just like we'd dreamed about in college.

On my twenty-third birthday, a few months before I needed to submit my application for the teaching program, I found myself in an hours-long conversation at a rooftop bar with the man who would become my boyfriend and then my husband.

Dan's life experiences were wildly different from mine: I had friends all over the country, planted in every town I'd called home, but my closest friends at the time were people I had known only a year or two. Dan's closest friends, on the other hand, were people he had known basically all his life. His college roommate was one of his childhood best friends, and his roommate at the time was another. While I'd started over with new people at a new school in a new state every few years, the only starting over Dan had done was moving down the street when he was not quite two years old.

By the time the teaching application deadline rolled around, I found myself pulled to stay put instead, to see whether our relationship would be worth it. I often questioned whether I was making the right decision. In some ways, staying home was the safer option compared to moving overseas indefinitely, but it felt risky to me—because I'd be staying for Dan. He represented the promise of interrupting my cycle of change, putting a stop to my life on the move, and settling me into a more permanent existence.

Choosing Dan was the first time I can remember choosing to live in and honor the present. After my first few childhood moves, I learned to look ahead to the next big thing, the next new place, the next time I could escape or make a change. Dan, however, is generally content wherever he is. His life has been marked by stability, and it shows in his quiet confidence, in his optimism, in his certainty that things will always work out for the best. I longed to give to my children this same stability. Through him, I began practicing the spiritual discipline of staying put, but I wanted my children to never have to learn it. Instead, I wanted it to be a way of life for our family.

As we packed up our apartment and prepared to move into the new house, I thought more concretely about the little one growing inside me. I instinctively wanted to protect him or her from the heartache I had experienced in childhood—a life on the move, frequent goodbyes, fighting to stay in the present, becoming addicted to change. My desire for this baby to know only one childhood home was an act of resistance, a way I could be different from my dad. His constant need for change had caused me pain and eventually trauma when he left our family to chase the next big thing.

Much of parenting seems to be centered on avoiding the mistakes our parents made. By parenting our children, we reparent ourselves too. If we grew up in a rigid, authoritarian household, we may swing the pendulum to the opposite approach and take on a child-centered parenting style. If we grew up in a home that felt disordered and chaotic, we may swing toward schedules and structure. If our parents pushed us to be high achievers, we may lower the bar for our kids; if our parents held low expectations for us, we may raise the bar. It's normal to want to give our kids the childhoods we wish we'd had.

Being pregnant brought my childhood experiences back to the surface as I thought about what I wanted to replicate and what I wanted to discard from my upbringing. As we slowly added furniture to our new home, I remembered the quintessentially '90s furniture that had accompanied my family through our every move: the navy-and-green plaid sofas, the burgundy gingham armchair, the TV with a built-in VCR. I used to cuddle on the sofa with my parents, watching Christmas movies as the snow fell outside. When I was sick, my mom would cover the sofa with old sheets, creating a makeshift bed in front of the TV. Other times, my siblings and I would pull the cushions off the furniture and scatter them across the floor; we leapt across them and tried not to fall into the "hot lava." This was something to retain: not just functional furniture built to withstand the force of children, but the feeling of coziness, security, and love the furniture represented.

The most important value in my childhood home was that my siblings and I were kind to each other with our words and bodies. My mom had grown up in a home where she and her siblings were allowed to fight physically. They would pull out each other's hair, scratch each other's eyes, and pin each other to the ground until the other person caved. In resistance, helping her children develop strong relationships to one another became her number-one goal. When we missed the mark, my parents showed us empathy and doled out fair and logical consequences. Like any child, I pushed against boundaries and believed my parents were horribly unfair, but I never felt disrespected or unsafe under their parenting style. This orientation toward empathy and relationships, then, was something to keep.

But the constant upheaval, the chase for new and bigger and better, the never-ending search for satisfaction—those things I wanted to discard.

Despite my true desires, I continued to feel the urge to move away and change things up. Days before we closed on our house, I somewhat jokingly asked Dan if we could forget it and move to Seattle instead. But each time that familiar feeling crept in, I recommitted to the things I wanted to be different for our family: stability of place, stability of purpose, stability of people.

As we consider the hopes and dreams we have for our growing families, we would do well to reflect on our own childhoods. What patterns do we still play out unintentionally, for better or for worse? What do we want to pass on to our children, and what do we want to spare them?

We carry our family histories in our muscle memory, but that does not mean we are beholden to them. Unexamined, unhealed history lodges itself inside of us as trauma, and it's hard, heavy work to make sense of it. But there is much we can glean from our stories, whether we do that introspection with a journal and a pen or with the help of a professional therapist. This is deeply creative and important work, fueling us to do better by our kids.

We won't get it all right, of course. Even children with the most loving, caring, empathetic parents don't escape childhood unscathed. By virtue of being human and living in the world, our children will experience pain. We as mothers are only human too—we do our best and fall short at times.

I don't say this to be fatalistic but to let us off the hook a bit.

Maybe the goal isn't to protect our children from all heartache and be perfect parents—though I'll bet many of us feel that instinct to our cores. Maybe a more accessible goal is to give our children the tools they need to face hardship and come out of it more resilient. And in whatever they may face, we can be a home base and stable place for our children to land.

10

Showing

"Hey, Dan, come look at this." I stood in our bathroom in front of the mirror, my shirt pulled up to reveal the bottom of my belly. "Do you think this is the baby or the burrito I ate for dinner?"

"You know, I think it's the baby this time."

I'd asked him some version of this question many times in the past few weeks, as I inspected my belly looking for signs of change. Until that point, whenever I noticed my abdomen was protruding more than usual, I concluded it was pregnancy-related bloating. But Google said I might start showing right around the second trimester, so that night I snapped a selfie—my first bump shot.

My Google search history at the time would have revealed questions like "What are the chances of miscarriage at five weeks?" and "Is it safe to take Tylenol in the first trimester?" and "Why can't I eat deli meat while pregnant?" Most of my questions were rooted in fear, but this one—"When will I start showing?"—was rooted in excitement. The prospect of watching my belly grow week by week, eventually filling out the stretchy panel of maternity pants, incited giddiness in me.

I was fascinated by pregnancy even as a child. I remember being at the grocery store with my mom when I was six years old, unable to take my eyes off a very pregnant woman in a floral maternity dress. I wondered how her belly could be so perfectly round since babies aren't shaped like basketballs. My mom became pregnant with my sister when I was eight, and she let press my hands to her belly as often as I wanted to. I was mesmerized by the baby's kicks and by the idea of another person being in there, someone I had never met but already loved.

A paradox of pregnancy is that it's both a deeply personal and an obtrusively public event. It usually begins with the most intimate, private act between two people, and then it develops within the private sphere of our bodies.

But as our bellies grow larger, our pregnancies become public knowledge—and simultaneously seem to invite unsolicited public commentary and, sometimes, unwanted public touch. There's something undeniably enchanting and almost invitational about a belly swelling with life and hope. (The key word here is "almost," because I think most pregnant women would agree that a baby bump is not actually an invitation for people to touch.)

I wanted my body to bear public witness to the miracle happening inside me, as if on some level I needed my still-imperceptible experience to be seen and acknowledged. In the most secret part of my heart, I wanted to feel like I was part of the club. I felt as though I'd waited forever after watching friend after friend become pregnant before I did, and I was eager for my turn to begin—at least in a visible way.

This child was already taking up a substantial chunk of my mind, energy, and love. I could sense in my heart what I was just beginning to feel in my body: every part of me was shifting to make space for a baby. My uterus was growing, pressing my intestines up and out of the way; my heart was expanding to hold love and responsibility for another human. My overwhelming desire was for this baby to continue to grow, to occupy my body and kick my ribs and leave me gasping for breath at the weight of it all—the weight of his or her body, the weight of the transformation I was undergoing, the weight of what was to come in motherhood.

And for the first time I could remember, my body seemed like a good and essential part of this spiritual change.

I grew up believing my flesh (meaning my body and my desires) was bad and not to be trusted, and the only thing I could truly trust was God's spirit. It led me to perceive, inaccurately, a division between the things of the body and the things of the soul, spirit, and heart. But the incarnation of Jesus obliterates that division. Through Jesus, God has a body—a body that existed first inside his mother and was fully dependent on her for nutrition and oxygen and protection.

God's chosen method of entering the world was through pregnancy and birth, which shows us that God identifies with our humanity in the most basic, concrete, embodied way. Jesus came into the world in a gush of water and blood from his mother's body, was wrapped in cloth and placed in his mother's arms, was nourished by her milk.

It leads me to wonder about Mary's experience with pregnancy. Did she worry about the safety of her child? Did she agonize over every decision, desiring first and foremost to keep him safe—not only because he was her son but also because he was the Son of God? Did Mary—a teenager pregnant with a baby that was not her husband's—place a hand on her belly as it started to swell, both in wonder and in dread, knowing she could not hide it from the public much longer?

Early in my church days, I learned that Jesus was both fully divine and fully human, but it strikes me now that his humanity was rarely emphasized. Occasionally I heard a sermon about how Jesus wept over the death of his friend Lazarus—a surprisingly human thing to do—or about the temptations of hunger and power he endured during his time in the wilderness. But I learned almost nothing about the miracle of Mary's pregnancy and Jesus's birth beyond the sanitized version of the Christmas story we read about in children's Bibles and hear preached by candlelight on Christmas Eve.

I heard little about the stories in the Bible where Jesus not only identifies with but *affirms* our humanity. Thomas, for example, didn't believe Jesus had been resurrected until he placed his own fingers into the nail holes in Jesus's hands. Whenever I've heard this story told, Thomas's doubts have been the focus—the message being that we shouldn't *need* to physically touch Jesus to believe in him. As I read the story now, what leaps off the page is the tenderness of Jesus, his deep understanding of Thomas's human nature, his validation of Thomas's humanity. Jesus invites him to verify the physicality of the resurrection by pressing the flesh of his own fingers against the flesh of Jesus's hands. Our spirituality is inextricably tied to our bodily experience, and it is good.

Thomas wasn't made to feel ashamed by his desire for embodied proof of a spiritual milestone. Likewise, most of us probably don't feel ashamed that we want our pregnant bellies to grow rounder and provide embodied proof of the spiritual change we're experiencing. I would imagine that many of us feel excitement as our bumps begin to pop out, perhaps even thinking, *Look, this is really happening! Look at what my body can do! Look at this miracle!*

Our growing bellies can certainly weigh us down and even cause deep pain and discomfort in the later stages of pregnancy, but they are first a source of grace. They are the evidence of this mysterious event we can't see, an event many of us have prayed and longed for.

They are the physical manifestation of the unseen processes unfolding in our bodies as we sustain the bodies of our children.

They are testaments to the lives we already love so deeply it might break us.

They are tangible talismans that ground us in the fact that we are changing and growing and stretching, that our bodies are wondrously making space for our babies and, in the process, transforming us into new versions of ourselves.

11

Eating for Two

Note: This chapter contains explicit details about my history with an eating disorder. I've included this story because I want to be honest about the ways in which I wrestled with my eating habits and body image in pregnancy. But I also want to be sensitive to readers who may be triggered by these topics. If this chapter will not be helpful at this point in your healing journey, please feel free to skip it.

As spring promised to become summer, I pulled my sundresses out of the closet to see which of them would work with my changing body. I assumed many of my dresses would fit differently but still be functional—perhaps even be cuter with a burgeoning bump underneath.

I wrestled myself into A-line floral prints, struggled with the straps of my favorite striped number, and tried to wiggle my hips into my standby black dress.

Nothing fit. *Not one thing.* Dresses that had once hung loosely on my frame now clung to my widening hips. My new flesh strained against the fitted waistlines, and for the first time in my life, I couldn't zip the dresses closed over my breasts. I was fascinated and delighted by my growing belly, but the changes everywhere else were unwelcome and left me feeling a little panicky.

I texted my two closest friends looking for solidarity in my shame, hiding my despair in self-deprecating humor and asking for advice on where to find cute maternity dresses. They came through, as they always do, but their pragmatic suggestions did nothing to quell the voice of my inner critic: *There are plenty of pregnant women out there who seem to be all belly. Why can't you be one of them?*

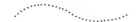

Body-image issues were nothing new to me at the age of twenty-eight. I had tried to lose weight for the first time when I was in seventh grade, which seems remarkably old given some of the statistics I've read: more than half of girls ages six to eight believe the ideal body is thinner than theirs, and one in four children has tried dieting by the time they turn seven.[4]

I was genuinely and blissfully unaware of my body in space—and in the eyes of others—until the summer I turned twelve. I wore the same lime-green bikini to the beach every weekend, but as the summer wore on, my body began to change, as is normal in adolescence: my abdomen softened and my thighs filled out. I had started that summer turning cartwheels on the beach, but I ended it sitting on the tailgate of my dad's truck, my arms wrapped around my growing waist in shame, confused about how quickly my body was changing compared to some of my friends'.

It was then that I began to view my body as the enemy, and I've spent much of my life frantically searching for a way to subdue it. For a long time, I thought there must be a single key that would unlock the perfect shape and ideal weight, along with all the ease that comes

---

4 Caitlin St John, "Body Image Issues Begin as Early as Age 5," *Parents*, accessed November 18, 2019, https://www.parents.com/health/parents-news-now/body-image-issues-begin-as-early-as-age-5.

with bodily perfection: Security! Happiness! A boy who would like me! Clothes that don't grow increasingly tight!

From the South Beach Diet to the paleo diet, from Tae Bo videos to marathon training, from cardio to strength, from bingeing to purging—I tried everything to make my body what I desired it to be.

My constant attempts to lose weight reached a dangerous low the spring after I broke up with my college boyfriend, Marshall. I knew I would be seeing him and his new girlfriend at a concert one Friday night, so the Monday before, I decided to do a five-day "experiment" (or, more accurately, "dangerous crash diet"). I would skip dinner every night that week in hopes of losing five pounds in five days.

Horrifyingly, it worked.

My jeans, usually a hair too snug, sat low on my hips that night as I danced along to the music, and I felt powerful and sexy and alive. The next morning, I logged my first long run of marathon-training season: eleven miles, faster than my usual pace.

My running was so strong, and the results of my experiment so deliciously addicting, that I decided to try it again the next week too, just to see whether I could lose ten pounds total and get down to my goal weight. To make faster progress, though, I upped the intensity by cutting out half my lunch.

But I didn't stop after week two.

As the weeks went by, I became trapped in a cycle of bingeing and purging. Instead of sticking my fingers down my throat, I slipped my feet into my running shoes and pounded the pavement harder and faster and longer than I had before. Somehow, while eating a dangerously small number of calories a day, I managed to run a personal-best time on a hilly half-marathon course. It was my proof that I was healthier than ever and in the best shape of my life.

Every weekend I was so hungry from my week of restriction and my Saturday long run that I would eat with abandon: pizza for lunch, a Frappuccino for a midday snack, brownies and cookies and canned frosting by the spoonful for dessert. I went out to dinner with friends, where we'd laugh over beers, burgers, and fries at our favorite gastro pubs. To everyone else, it looked like I was living in freedom. But I was a slave to the scale and the constant tightening of my pants.

Every week, I would lose five pounds, and every weekend, I would gain it back, plus some.

I drove myself mad wondering why, even though I was eating less and working out more than I ever had, I couldn't seem to lose weight and keep it off. I weighed myself every morning and tried on my smallest pair of jeans every night, examining myself in the mirror and determining whether I had more or less muffin top than I'd had the day before. My inner critic never missed an opportunity to berate me: *Your jeans feel tight because you ate nine pretzels at lunch today instead of eight. Everyone is going to notice the extra flesh on your arms at the beach this weekend. You should run harder during your workout tomorrow.*

About eight weeks into this extreme weight-loss attempt, my body gave out, and I injured my knee in the middle of marathon training. It was devastating at the time, but looking back, I realize how lucky I was that nothing worse happened. I visited my primary care doctor to get a prescription for physical therapy, and at the end of the appointment, she asked whether I had any other concerns or questions about my health.

"Actually, I do," I began. "For the past few months I've been cutting calories and running more, but I seem to be gaining weight. Is there anything else I can do to get my weight under control?"

With compassion and perhaps some trepidation in her voice, she asked me, "Can you tell me more about the measures you're taking? What do you eat, and how much are you running?"

I told her everything. On some level I think I wanted to be found out—for someone to see how much agony I was in and how unhealthy my life had become. It was better for that intervention to come from someone with an objective perspective, as I likely would have become defensive if a loved one had tried to help me see the truth.

The doctor explained that what I was doing was unhealthy at best and dangerous at worst. She referred me not just to physical therapy for my knee but also to a dietician to help me get back on a healthy-for-me eating plan and to a therapist to help me process the emotional side of what I was going through. She warned me that I would likely gain more weight before my body finally leveled out, but that it was a necessary part of the healing process. I had traumatized my body, and now it needed sustenance and permission to reshape itself.

Utterly exhausted from the way I was living, I complied. I scheduled weekly appointments with the dietician, followed her advice, and put on twenty pounds to prove it. I knew I had to keep going, but even so, I cried every time I stepped on the scale and every time I outgrew a pair of pants, blaming myself and feeling completely powerless.

Regardless of how much or how little weight we gain during pregnancy, it's a jarring experience to live in a body that is changing so rapidly. In the span of less than a year, our bodies become almost unrecognizable: larger limbs, wider hips, new stretch marks, a belly that becomes so big and round that we can't see our feet or shave our legs or turn over in the night without grunting and breaking a sweat.

Being pregnant triggered the same powerless feeling I had when I was gaining weight during my eating-disorder recovery, the same sensation that I was a stranger in my own body. In both situations, the weight gain was necessary for my health and well-being. Yet in both situations, I resisted my body and experienced intense frustration and shame that I couldn't make it behave.

On the late-spring day when I discovered none of my dresses fit my changing figure, Dan came home from work and found me in the wreckage of our closet. I let loose on him all the venom that had built within me, whispered in my ear by that awful inner voice.

"Nothing fits! Look at this dress—it was so big on me when I bought it last winter that I thought about having it tailored. Now I can't even zip it up! And look at the way this one clings. It used to be my favorite dress." I took a breath and continued, my voice cracking with emotion: "Have you seen my thighs? My hips? I don't even recognize myself. I've seen so many pregnant women on Instagram who seem to be getting bigger only in their bellies. Why can't I be like them?"

By this point, Dan was used to my struggle: we had started dating at the height of my recovery weight gain, and he had seen me fall prey to the insidious thinking again. In the two years we'd been married, I had done multiple Whole30s and tried new workout programs and skipped dessert for weeks at a time in an effort to maintain the weight I'd been at our wedding. (Nothing worked.) Most of the time he was sensitive and supportive, but on this day, his frustration flared.

"I really want to help you, but it's so hard to listen to this same negative talk every day. I want to see you be *happy* with your body. I want you to be healthy and strong. But you're obsessed, and it's hard to watch. It kills me to see you living with regret every time you eat something unhealthy or your jeans get a little tight." He sighed and then continued, "I wish you could see your body for what it is: *it's normal.*"

"It's normal, but it's not perfect," I retorted.

"No, it's not. And neither is mine. I don't know anyone in real life who has a perfect body."

The tension drained from his voice as he added this: "Look, what if this baby is a girl? Are you going to let her see you struggle like this? Do you really want to pass this on to her? I know you'd try to hide it and stop her from seeing how you treat yourself. But she'll know."

She'll know.

I sank onto our bed, struggling under the weight of his words. For the first time in my life, it wasn't just *my* body I was responsible for. When I was in the throes of disordered eating, it was I who paid the price: *my* knee got injured, *my* hair fell out, *my* face exploded with acne—all the result of choices I had made that threw my body into a state of panic.

But now I was carrying a child, and my eating choices directly impacted him or her. Restricting myself now held real consequences for another person. And even though all the pregnancy books told me exactly which foods to eat to ensure the baby would be as healthy as possible, I knew adhering to any sort of dieting rules could send me into dangerous territory with my mental and physical health—and my baby's too.

It wouldn't end when the baby was born, either. Postpregnancy life wouldn't hand me a free pass to become a fitness fanatic and a healthy-eating junkie again. Little eyes would notice and try to make sense of what Mommy was doing. A little heart would absorb the value I placed on appearance and would learn to prize it above all else.

I knew what I needed to do: resist my inner critic instead of resisting my body.

It was overwhelming to face down the critical voice I had lived with my whole life. I failed often. I beat myself up when I gained more than the recommended one pound a week, and I felt ashamed every time I outgrew a maternity shirt that had once been too big for me.

But when it comes to progress, especially in changing our thought patterns, there is no finish line. All we can do is take one small step at a time and believe it will add up to real change someday. If a tiny trickle of water can carve away stone, then surely changing one thought at a time can chip away at even a lifetime of negative self-perception.

My first step had been giving myself permission to eat chips for dinner. My subsequent steps could be just as small: ordering my favorite French toast at brunch; asking the nurse not to tell me my weight at my final few doctor's appointments; declaring at a few weeks postpartum that I didn't care at all whether I lost the baby weight—and actually meaning it. (Eventually, I did care, but I made progress again when I settled into a bigger size than I had been before and decided it was my new normal.)

I still take steps backward when I accidentally make comments about my weight in front of my child, but I inch forward every time I affirm my little one's strength and intellect and sense of humor—and when I affirm my own strengths in range of those listening ears.

If you find yourself stuck in a pattern of taking too many steps backward, of feeling bad about yourself and wishing your body were different, consider talking to yourself the way you would talk to your dearest friend. What would you say to her about her pregnant body? What would you want her to believe about herself? And why would you want her to believe it? I would imagine you'd tell her she's valuable at any size, in any stage of life, because she is *herself*. You wouldn't say it to coddle her or simply to make her feel better—you'd say it because you genuinely mean it, and you want her to believe it too.

As we practice speaking words of grace to ourselves, may we come to know, deep in our bones, both that our bodies are important—we couldn't be pregnant or savor our favorite foods or relish a touch from our loved ones without them—and that we are so much more than what our bodies look like or how much space they take up.

When I was eight years old, I attended Take Our Daughters and Sons to Work Day with a close family friend. I don't remember now what her job title was or what her company did. What I do remember is the way she walked down the hall. I noticed the way her body moved through space, how she took up as much room as she needed. Her legs were sturdy and sure as her heels thudded against the carpet.

My eight-year-old brain scanned for the right word to describe what I was seeing. I landed on this thought: *Wow, she's so skinny.*

But this woman was not "skinny."

The word my brain couldn't locate was *powerful*. She was *powerful*.

At that young age, I had already equated power with the size of a woman's body. I had already started to believe that the most important thing a woman can be is small and that she is at the height of her power when she takes up the least amount of space.

Let's declare this together now: *This will not be true for our children.*

May our children always know the word *powerful*.

May they always know *they* are powerful.

May they always know power is a gift to be wielded carefully and for good.

And may we demonstrate what power looks like by taking up all the space we need in the world.

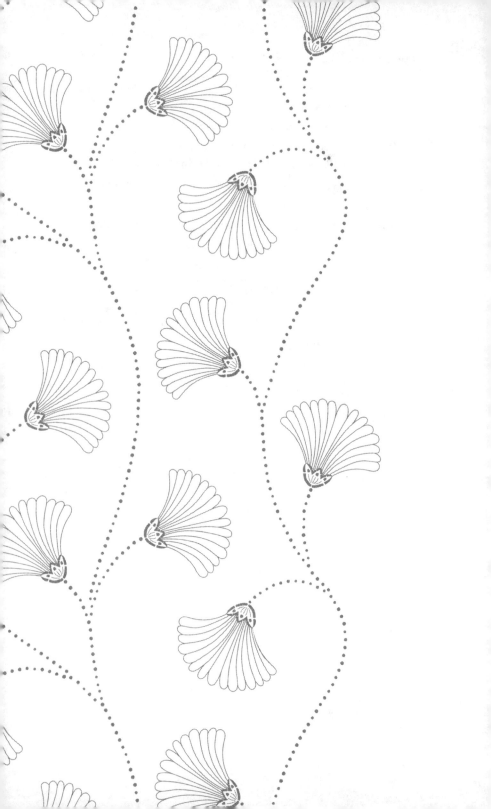

The Sisterhood of the Full-Panel Jeans

12

Maternity clothes are quite possibly the greatest perk of pregnancy, and yet I avoided wearing them at first because of my deep-seated body-image issues. I had wanted to wear my regular clothes as long as possible, as if doing so would mean I was gaining weight and getting bigger only in my belly (which was entirely not true).

More quickly than I could have imagined, my jeans became intolerable. The thighs were too tight, and I wore the waistbands unzipped and stretched as wide as they could go, using a belly band to hold them up. I struggled and wrestled my way into my pants every morning, and afterward I felt like a stuffed sausage. When I could no longer handle the discomfort of my jeans button digging into my skin, I caved and asked my mom to help me pick out some maternity clothes.

We met at an outdoor mall on a warm June afternoon. Bold pink and orange flowers spilled out of cement planters. The sunshine was welcome after a long winter and rainy spring; even the sweat that formed along my hairline was an exciting sign of seasonal change.

We stepped into the maternity clothing store, where I tried on jeans with hidden elastic waistbands, side panels, demi panels, and full panels; tops with empire waists and side ruching; dresses that tied in the back and had extra fabric in the front. As I pulled on each item, stretching them over my belly, I discovered the best-kept secret of pregnancy: maternity clothes are *magic*.

For so long, I had felt constant pressure to hide my imperfections under my clothes, but suddenly my growing midsection was something to celebrate rather than conceal. Maternity clothes seemed uniquely designed to enhance instead of camouflage, to provide comfort and support instead of shame. As I gazed at myself in the dressing-room mirror, I wished that all women's clothing, maternity and not, could be this gentle on our bodies.

With a shopping bag in each hand, I returned home and hung up my finds in the closet, resolving to wear only maternity clothes from that day forward. Rather than a concession to my inability to restrain my growing body, this decision was a way to show myself compassion and claim the space I needed. My body and my spirit melted into the softness of my new clothing. Instead of stuffing myself into pieces that weren't made for this season of my body's life, I slipped on material that gently stretched with me—that made way for this baby, my new body, and my changing identity.

When we experience a significant emotional event—receive devastating news, witness an emergency, or experience deep surprise—we often develop a flashbulb memory. We can recall the moment in incredible, vivid detail: where we were sitting, who we were with, what the air smelled like, what we were wearing. Pregnancy seems to intensify everything else in our lives, adding weight and significance to things we may not have thought much about otherwise. We undergo a remarkable amount of change in a short span of time, and I think because of this, we create mini flashbulb memories throughout these nine months.

Each article of my maternity clothing represents one of those moments. The dresses and jeans and tops connect me to that tender time, each one bringing me right back to a specific memory—either of pregnancy or of regular life that kept happening all around me, even as I was undergoing this transformation.

There was the navy-and-white striped dress I wore on my twenty-eighth birthday, when Dan and I went out for brunch and then shopped for a rug to place in our new home. The year before, my birthday had fallen on a day of uncertainty: it was my last day of work after quitting my job, and I didn't have another one lined up. But since that birthday, I had found a job I loved, and we had also bought a house and adopted a dog. As we browsed rugs and talked about our avocado-sized baby growing beneath the ruching of my dress, barely visible to anyone but us, I felt sure and steady.

The first maternity top that fit me when I was barely showing was a short-sleeved V-neck tee made of slub cotton with thin pink and white stripes. I wore it the night we found out our baby's sex and during a trip to Colorado with my college friends. Their hands had once held mine as we watched sappy movies in our dorm rooms; they had petted my hair while I cried over breakups that really were for the best, even if I couldn't see it at the time. And years later, these friends rested their hands on my belly, waiting for the flutter of a little foot.

I was twenty-four weeks pregnant when my brother got married—not far enough along to feel uncomfortably large but far enough to be surprised at how much I had changed. I wore a gray knee-length chiffon dress with a deep V and a single ruffle that ran across the front. The silky fabric swished across my legs as I danced that night, and there was plenty of room for me to eat two pieces of cake.

By the time I hit thirty-seven weeks, I wanted nothing to do with the fitted maternity clothes I'd loved in the beginning. While I had once relished how they showed off my growing belly, I now felt itchy and confined within them. I switched them out for the oversized, super-soft T-shirts a friend had lent me, paired with a revolving collection of maternity yoga pants that I had stretched about as far as the waistbands would allow. The last few weeks of my pregnancy were full of tension and anxiety and illness, and these gentle clothes were a tactile way I could care for myself.

Months after my child was born—many more months than I had expected—I folded each item of maternity clothing and placed them all in a long plastic bin, storing the clothes and the memories under my bed for safekeeping until I would need them again.

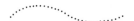

One March weekend after I'd had the baby, my next-door neighbor, Alyssa, texted to see whether Dan and I wanted to meet her and her husband, Matt, at the dog park. We loaded up our four-month-old and our dog, Riley, and made the short drive there. I strapped the baby into the carrier, and we set off.

I was eager to see Alyssa. We hadn't talked in a few weeks—not because we were too busy, but because I was giving her some space. She and her husband had been walking through the IVF process for months, and four weeks earlier, she'd finally been able to undergo the transfer procedure. At the time, she described how she watched on the ultrasound monitor as the doctor inserted the embryo into her uterus—a tiny bubble, a real life. She walked out of the office that day with her baby inside her but would have to wait a week before finding out if the embryo had implanted successfully. She would take a pregnancy test at her doctor's office the following Friday, and I assured her I wouldn't text her to ask about the results. She could let me know her news, for better or for worse, whenever she was ready.

Days had turned into weeks, and I ached for her, hoping her silence was a sign of happy news, and maybe she was waiting to clear some milestone before sharing. I prayed for her most nights, asking God to comfort her in her pain and longing if she wasn't pregnant, or to protect her and fill her with joy if her baby was indeed growing.

As Alyssa and Matt approached us at the park, I scanned her face for any indication of what had happened, feeling insecure about the baby strapped to my chest, a reminder of what I had that she longed for. She glanced at Matt for a moment and then told us she was pregnant and due in November. I squealed and congratulated her with a hug, and then I started firing the usual questions: "How are you feeling? Any nausea? Who have you told?"

We grimaced together as we talked about her morning sickness and exhaustion, acknowledging what a pain and a relief it is to have such a tangible reminder of the life growing inside. We discussed bloating and showing, and projected when her belly would start to pop.

I offered to let her borrow my maternity clothes, and when I brought them to her later that week, it felt as if I were extending her an invitation to experience the magic.

Since then, I've lent these clothes out to another dear friend, Stephanie. She was pregnant with her first after a long period of waiting and wondering and wishing. These clothes—the soft jeans and striped shirts and flowy tanks—have grown and stretched with three women, made room for three new people in this world, and knitted us together in the process. Each piece came back to me carrying a new set of memories: moments of worry and relief, sorrow and celebration, loneliness and belonging.

I pulled the clothes out from under my bed a few years later, anticipating I would need them again after getting a positive pregnancy test. I had long hoped my body would require these clothes a second time; that I would carry another life and experience the rapid expansion of my belly and my heart; that I would hang these pieces in my closet again, each one filled with my memories and those of my friends as well. But before I even had a chance to wash them, I began to bleed.

I had expected to share my happy news with Alyssa and Stephanie, but instead I had to find the words to say I'd had a miscarriage. In the aftermath, they checked on me, provided dinner, offered to care for my first child while I recovered, and reminded me to care for myself and not be too quick to jump back into regular life.

I did become pregnant again, and this time, Alyssa lent me her maternity clothes to supplement my own. Stephanie surprised me with a Target gift card as a way of saying thank you, so I could replace the jeans that had become worn out from all the growth they'd seen.

When I finally had the chance to slip those clothes back on, it was like a reunion. They were softer than ever, ready to embrace me as I processed all that had happened since the last time I saw them, ready to stretch alongside me as I became a mom all over again.

It goes without saying that our bodies and souls need support as we become mothers, but perhaps support can come in ways we never expected. Maybe you'll find it in a borrowed pair of jeans that make you feel confident and alive in your changing state. Maybe you'll find it in a flowy floral dress, worn by multiple moms celebrating at their baby showers. Maybe it will show up as a box on your front porch, filled with hand-me-down nursing tops.

Wherever that provision comes from, I hope it will point to a community of fellow mothers who will carry you through the hardest moments of carrying a child, who will remind you to be brave and compassionate toward yourself. And I hope when your body and soul have come to rest in their new shape, you will pay the magic forward.

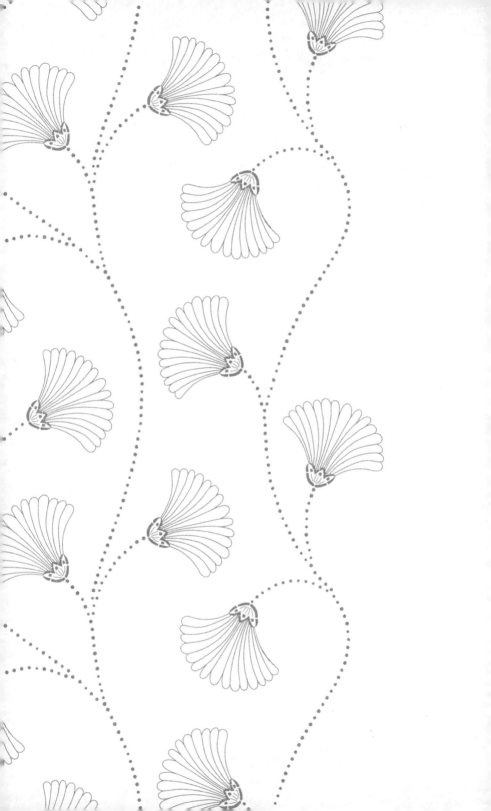

13

It's A...

When Dan and I decided to start a family, I not-so-secretly dreamed of having a blond-haired, blue-eyed little girl who looked like me. It strikes me now as a silly or even selfish wish, but I think this is human nature: we want to live on somehow, whether through our children or through some other legacy, such as achievement or art.

I've always been "girly" myself, at least in some ways—I refused pants in favor of dresses for my entire kindergarten career (this became a problem in Chicago's subzero winter weather), chose bubblegum-pink carpeting for my first big-girl room, and loved hair bows all the way through college. As I've grown into adulthood, I've come to understand that the expectations we place on girls to perform femininity in a certain way can be harmful. There's no right way to be feminine. Even still, I continue to love pink and frills.

I longed for a girl because I wanted to buy all those pink, frilly things for a tiny person. I imagined pink footie pajamas, ruffle-bottomed leggings, and a rainbow assortment of hair bows and headbands. I pictured snuggling her in a pink nursery and carefully styling her pigtails. Of course, I believe that any child of mine can be exactly who they want to be and express their gender however feels right to them. But if I did have a girl, then at least for her first couple of years, I'd be able to indulge my affection for baby-girl gear.

For much of my first trimester, I didn't have a strong inkling about our baby's sex, but I tended to believe it was male. Nearly all my friends had children at this point, and nearly all those children were girls, so statistically, it made sense that there wouldn't be another one in our bunch. Each baby has a fifty-fifty shot, but what were the odds that so many of them would be biologically female?

In a way, I was bracing myself for the idea that this baby could be a boy. If I wanted a girl and believed it was a girl, I'd surely get my hopes too high. If mitigating disappointment is all about managing expectations, then I would expect a boy. I was certain I would be utterly smitten with whoever our baby turned out to be, but I was also afraid—not of having a boy, but of being *disappointed* that I was having a boy, even if the disappointment lasted only a moment. I didn't want to have to come around to the idea of my child's sex or pin my hopes on any one trait—I wanted to love everything about him or her from the very beginning.

I also knew how complicated gender is and that it's not always tied to sex. But I was doing my best to make sense of my child's identity with the limited information I had access to during pregnancy, before I could really know who he or she would turn out to be.

Somewhere around the beginning of the second trimester, a switch flipped in my gut, and I knew I was having a girl. To this day, I'm not sure what changed or whether this was mother's intuition (for all I knew, I could be completely wrong). But one day I went from thinking the baby might be a boy to *knowing* I was carrying a girl.

As I counted down the weeks to my twenty-week ultrasound, I felt like a small child waiting for Christmas: eager with anticipation, giddy at the prospect of unwrapping a precious gift, and uneasy at the thought of being disappointed. Though I was eager to find out the baby's sex, I was equally excited to get to see our baby for the first time since week eight, when he or she was a jelly bean with arms and legs. This time, our little one would have a developed profile and body, functioning organs, and individual fingers and toes.

My bump was growing seemingly by the day; I was feeling kicks with increasing regularity and intensity; I had heard the heartbeat strong and clear at every doctor's appointment. But getting to see my baby's face—even if it was just a projection of sound, the resulting image grainy and gray—was a new and thrilling level of connection.

The day of the ultrasound, I went to work as usual and met Dan at the doctor's office over my lunch break. As I shifted restlessly in my chair, I noticed only a mild sense of anxiety about the appointment, despite it being a major anatomy scan. In my eagerness to find out the baby's sex, I'd almost forgotten that the doctor had a much bigger and more important purpose for this appointment than seeing my child's button nose or announcing whether it was a boy or a girl. This felt like a testament to how much I'd grown not just physically but emotionally during pregnancy: my first-trimester self would have been terrified about this appointment, envisioning all the things that could go wrong and rehearsing how to receive bad news. Instead, today seemed like just another fun milestone.

As I waited for the nurse to call my name, I placed a hand on my belly, closed my eyes, and thought of my friends who had received unexpected or devastating news at these appointments. I asked God to be near to us whatever the outcome, whether we received joyful news that all was well or crushing news that something was wrong.

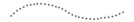

After a longer wait than expected—made even longer because of my restless energy—Dan and I were finally guided to the ultrasound room. I maneuvered myself onto the table, the paper crinkling under me to announce my every move. The darkness of the room, the glow of blue lights on the screen, and the low hum of the machines brought me straight back to the first scan, when I thought I was miscarrying. My eyelids fluttered closed, and I felt the deep contrast between the sharpness of my fear that day and the buoyancy of the optimism welling up in me now.

The technician helped me get situated and then squirted my belly with the ultrasound gel, cold enough to make me gasp and cause my hair to prickle. She placed the wand firmly against my skin, and where there had once been a blank screen, the form of a baby—*my child*—materialized.

She navigated the wand around my belly, clicking computer keys to zoom in on the baby's face and pointing out the nose, jawline, and mouth. My whole body began to shake with laughter, also shaking up the image, and I apologized as joyful tears slid down my cheeks. Dan squeezed my hand as we gazed in wonder at the little life who was right there with us, present in that very room, making a home in my body. He or she had been there all along, but the realization of this child's embodiment washed over us in a fresh way as we watched our little one blow tiny bubbles and suck their thumb.

Awestruck, we whispered over and over, "There's our baby."

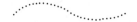

At the end of the ultrasound, the technician gave us the customary prints—one of our baby's tiny feet, one of the whole body, and one of the profile. Later, I would hang the images on our refrigerator door, where they'd remain for the rest of my pregnancy. We'd told the technician at the beginning of the appointment that we wanted to know the baby's sex but wanted to find out over dinner later, so she handed me a sealed envelope containing the information, asked with a sly smile whether I could be trusted with it, and then wished us well.

Dan and I emerged into the sunshine, reliving and replaying the highlights of the past hour. "Can you believe we could see all the toes?" "Didn't the baby look strong?" "Do you think the shape of the baby's head is normal? It's probably normal." (It was normal.)

We agreed to leave the envelope in the trunk of my car, and I promised a dozen times that I wouldn't peek.

The rest of the day moved in a strange time warp, minutes becoming hours and hours becoming days, and I had to get up to pee more times than I could count. When I finally left work, I called Dan to tell him we wouldn't be wasting any time—he should be ready to get in the car and head to dinner as soon as I got home. We had decided to celebrate at our favorite restaurant and order our favorite thing on the menu: pulled-pork nachos with homemade barbecue sauce and plenty of sliced jalapeños.

After the waiter disappeared with our order, we pulled out the envelope—the one containing the information that, while not exactly life changing, I'd been pining for since the moment I found out I was pregnant. Dan scooted around to my side of the booth, and I broke the seal and pulled out a folded notecard.

We both took a deep breath, and as I gently lifted the corner of the card, I saw the smallest glimpse of pink, and a squeal sprang from my mouth. Dan popped the card open the rest of the way, confirming the details: inside were the words "It's a girl!" in white block letters against a pink background. He wrapped me in a tight hug, as much as the booth would allow, and I dissolved into a fit of giggles and tears, overjoyed at the idea of having a girl—my little girl.

As Dan slid back into his side of the booth, I remembered our daughter already had a name.

"We're having a Selah!" I told him as I laughed and dabbed my eyes with a napkin. Though we hadn't agreed on anything for a boy, we had chosen this girl name long before I even got pregnant.

As realization washed over him too, his smile spread and his eyes crinkled as he repeated my words, whispering, "We're having a Selah."

Speaking her name aloud for the first time, assigning it to her and affirming that she was chosen and known and named, was a crystallizing moment for me: God had known this child from the very start—her sex, her name, her every detail. And God knew how this child would grow and change and express her gender identity in the future, the talents she would possess, the things that would bring her joy, and the work that would light her on fire. Not only that, but God was entrusting her life to *us*. The pain and the worry, the joy and the excitement, the anxiety and the uncertainty I'd felt for the past twenty weeks all converged in a single breath: *Selah*.

As the news began to sink in, Dan looked at me with less sparkle and more seriousness in his eyes as he said, "You know, we're not just having a little girl. We'll be raising a teenage daughter."

The weight of what we were in for began to settle in my chest, not in an entirely unwelcome way but in the way little white flakes settle at the bottom of a snow globe. I added on to his thought: "Not only that. We'll be shaping a *woman*."

Suddenly my excitement over a prospective mini me, one I could dress in pink and go on mommy-daughter dates with, began to feel something more like a commissioning. I wasn't just being given a chance to outfit a little girl; I was being given a chance to raise up a woman. I didn't know whether she'd be introverted like me or extroverted like her dad, whether she'd be sweet or spicy, amiable or feisty, cautious or fearless, thoughtful or impulsive, an artist or an intellectual or both. But I knew in my bones, in my blood, in my whole being that I'd do everything I could to help her know herself and be herself and love herself.

In a time of life when we are preparing for all things baby and trying to make sense of what's coming, we can easily (and understand-ably) forget that our children won't be babies forever. The baby stage is an important but remarkably small part of raising humans through adulthood. Our children may land anywhere on the gender spectrum, have a wide variety of personality traits and talents and passions, and will change and grow for the rest of their lives.

Despite the details of who our children turn out to be, I would guess many of us have common goals: We want to raise children who become kind and brave and honest adults. We want them to become people who act with integrity and radiate joy and admit when they're wrong and learn from their mistakes. People who are gracious with themselves and therefore with others. People who know how loved they are, who love themselves because they know they carry God's image, who recognize God in everyone they meet, who extend love and compassion and empathy because of this.

Perhaps we as parents are less like sculptors—deciding who our children should be and then chiseling and shaping them until we deem them finished.

Perhaps we are more like road maps, showing our children the available routes to becoming who God planned for them to be all along.

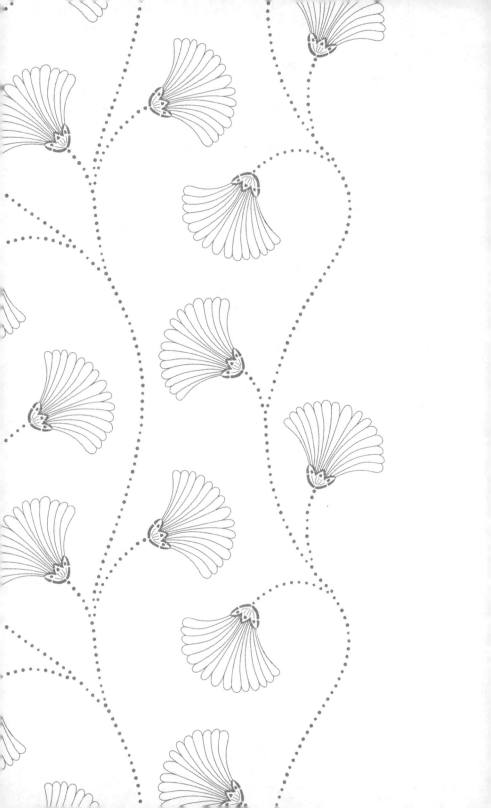

14

Baby Registry

An icy blast of air conditioning rushed over my skin as the sliding doors closed behind me and Dan, sealing us into another world. Towering product displays and bright lights assaulted my vision, and the ceilings were so tall it felt as if we had stepped into a warehouse. Boxes filled with bottles and bedding and baby toys were stacked precariously high along every wall.

I took a deep breath and clutched my printed spreadsheet a little tighter.

It was time to take on the big-box baby store.

I'd been inside this colossal store a few times before to pick up registry gifts for friends, and every time, I'd had the sense that I didn't belong. The floor layout confused me, and I didn't know what half the products were used for. On this day, I still felt confused and over-whelmed by the immensity of the store and the amount I didn't know—but this time I felt as though I was supposed to be here. I had a little one flipping around inside me, and I was about to use all my pent-up planning energy to choose baby items for her.

We stepped over to the registry counter, where a bubbly woman welcomed us and told us to take a seat in the chairs in front of her desk. She began peppering us with questions: "When are you due?" "Do you know if it's a boy or a girl?" "Are you sharing the gender on your registry?"

After she entered all our personal information into her computer and officially set up our registry, she handed us a scanner gun and a brochure with a list of suggested items in each category—feeding, diapering, and baby gear, just to start—and then set us loose.

"Wait, isn't someone going to walk around with us?" I asked, my voice betraying a mild sense of alarm.

I remembered back to the day when Dan and I registered for our wedding at a similar store. An overeager employee had walked us through every department and decision—and I had already possessed a working knowledge of china and cutting boards and coffee makers. All these baby gadgets felt like tools from a different time and place, entirely foreign to me. I needed a guide.

"So sorry!" the registry assistant exclaimed with a bright smile. "We're short staffed today, so you'll have to get started on your own. But if you have any questions, there should be someone on the floor who can help you. We always have someone on duty in strollers if you want to start there."

I thanked her and stood up, turning to Dan with a fake-it-till-you-make-it sense of confidence. I had come to the store equipped with a printed spreadsheet of registry favorites from a popular baby-product review site, all organized by category and price point. I figured I would start with the recommendations for a given item, expand my visual search of the department to make sure I didn't like anything else better, swiftly and decisively choose a product, and then move on to the next thing on the list. How complicated could it be?

Thanks to my research and input from friends, I had already narrowed my search to three strollers. With the promise of finding a set of helping hands in that department, I marched over with Dan trailing behind.

"Let's try out the models I'm interested in. If there's one that clearly folds and unfolds easier than the others, let's go with that one," I told him.

The on-the-floor employee was swamped working with three other couples, so we started exploring on our own. Twenty minutes later, we hadn't found the models I was looking for and instead were pulling out random strollers and testing them. Not a single one worked intuitively—we even had to leave a few models folded up because we couldn't figure out how to pop them back open.

We had two hours available before Dan had to go to work, and even though I knew we wouldn't be able to knock out the whole registry in that timeframe, I also didn't want to spend all our time in one department. I suggested we proceed to something easier and less expensive: diaper bags.

Once again, I could not find the exact bags on my list, so I started picking up bags that caught my eye, unzipping pouch after pouch and imagining what I might need to place inside each one.

"What do you think of this pattern?" I asked Dan about a gray bag printed with white damask scrolls.

"I'd carry it, but it's a little boring. What about something more colorful?"

(This sums up our approach to home decor too. I'm drawn to soft neutrals and believe gray is a pop of color. Dan, on the other hand, loves variety and vibrance, words that have never once been used to describe my taste.)

We examined at least a dozen other diaper bags, which were just a fraction of the bags on display, stacked on shelves higher than we could reach. The interior pockets in each model were set in slightly different places, this one offering an insulated bottle pouch but that other one boasting a cell phone pocket. Some were messenger style, some backpack style, some hybrid. Most had fold-out changing pads, but a few didn't, and there were portable changing pads available for purchase separate from the bags.

Fifteen more minutes had gone by, and I felt no closer to making a decision as the options began to run together in one murky current through my mind.

"I don't want to spend all our time here either!" I finally said. I was teetering on the edge between exasperation and panic over a diaper bag—which felt more than justified at the time. I felt an intense pressure to pick the exact right bag, right now, for all time. "Let's scan these three. I remember liking them, but I don't remember why. I'll do more research and read reviews at home and then pick one."

We agreed to move on to something even less expensive and more basic: crib sheets and mattress pads. They all function essentially the same way, and picking out sheets was just a matter of taste. Easy.

We asked an employee to direct us toward the bedding, thinking it would be a semicontained department like the strollers and bags.

"You can find it all along the back wall, organized by brand, not by type of item."

My head began to spin as I took in the reality of the situation. The entire back wall of the store? It appeared to be about the length of a city block. *Point me toward the most basic mattress pads!* I thought. *I want those!*

Dan and I started at one end of the massive wall, our eyes scanning up and down, trying to glance at each product before continuing.

I dismissed each package of sheets Dan pointed out: "I'd prefer polka dots, not stripes." "Nothing with butterflies." "Those colors are too bright." "Those are a little too plain." Dan was growing irritated—a small sigh here, a check of his phone there. At one point he started voice-dictating an email to a client, and I lost it: "Do you even want to be here?"

"Honestly? Not anymore. This whole process is overwhelming, and you seem to have a vision in your head that I'm not in on, and we're not getting anything done."

"Let's leave then," I muttered. "I'll do it all online."

Tears began to stream down my face as we walked out of the store. A tense silence filled the space between us, replacing the shared eagerness we'd come in with. I pecked Dan goodbye, got into my car, and then posted a desperate plea for registry advice on Facebook.

I felt silly for being so upset over a baby registry—but I also felt an undeniable pressure to get it "right." These strollers, car seats, and carriers were the devices I would use to restrain my child and rely on to keep her safe. The bottles I chose would either support my breastfeeding goals or work against them. The toys I picked would either be safe or unsafe, helpful or harmful to my baby's brain development. Some crib mattresses were linked to greater rates of sudden infant death syndrome, but those that weren't cost three times as much.

Every decision felt like a matter of life or death, or least of safety or danger. If I couldn't choose the right baby items for my registry, what hope would I have of being a mom who could actually *use* these items to care for her baby? Really, what kind of mom can't even fold and unfold a stroller?

Quicker than I expected, my mom friends came to the rescue in the comments on my post:

"I totally understand. I had a similar experience when we went to register for Will. I was so overwhelmed and felt like maybe I was going to have a panic attack, so we left, consulted parents in the know, and did the online route."

"Yeah, it's a little overwhelming! I walked through the store with my sister when she registered, and I like to think it helped her. Let me know if you want to wander the aisles with me!"

"Oh friend, I feel you! I took a mom friend with me who has three littles so she could tell me what to actually get. It was super helpful!"

And finally: "I totally understand this! Besides a place for the baby to sleep and a car seat, I figured out everything else along the way. It's such a personal thing and what you need is different for each mama!"

I had wanted to pick exactly the right items that would guarantee my baby's safety and happiness. I've always hated the process of trial and error—I prefer to get it right the first time, and if I don't, I'm embarrassingly quick to give up. But these messages were the permission slip I needed both to be overwhelmed and to not take this baby-registry thing so seriously.

So what if I didn't know how to use a NoseFrida? So what if I changed my mind about a diaper bag a few months into parenting? So what if my baby hated the swaddle blankets I chose—blankets that were just the right intersection of breathable and cute?

None of it would have any bearing on my ability to be a good mom—that's what.

None of it has any bearing on your ability to be a good mom either. Our baby-registry skills say nothing about our moral character or maternal instincts.

We know that adding babies to our families and becoming moms for the first time will change our lives completely—but it's impossible to know what the change will be like until we experience it. We can try to be as prepared as possible, which is not a bad impulse, but it can lead us to put pressure on things that aren't terribly important, simply because they are things we can plan for now and take with us into the next phase. The bottles we buy now will accompany us into new motherhood, as will the crib and the diapers and the stroller.

But that stuff is not what makes us mothers.

We will hold those bottles. We will gently lay our babies in their cribs. We will tirelessly wipe their bottoms seventeen times a day or push them around in their strollers when they won't sleep any other way. The fact that we want to choose all the "right" products reveals that our hearts are in the right place, even if our actions are a bit misguided. We already want to do what's best for our kids.

But here's the thing: our babies will have needs and desires and preferences we can't predict. They don't come to us as blank slates, ready to enjoy the pacifiers we painstakingly picked or the diapers we thought would prevent both leaks and rashes. Perhaps we can't anticipate their needs now, but we can trust that we'll recognize them when our babies present them. And for the things we can't quite figure out—when he has leaked through three kinds of diapers or she seems to hate every pacifier ever made—we can lean on friends who have done this before, and then someday, we can share our hard-earned wisdom with other new moms.

We'll make plenty of mistakes, of course—on our registries and in the day-to-day of mothering. Taking risks and making mistakes and learning lessons again and again are part of the deal with parenting, even for those of us who would rather get everything right the first time.

So whichever products you pick, remember that each item is simply a tool in your loving hands. You can let go of the goal to nail the perfect registry because ultimately, what's best for your baby is *you*.

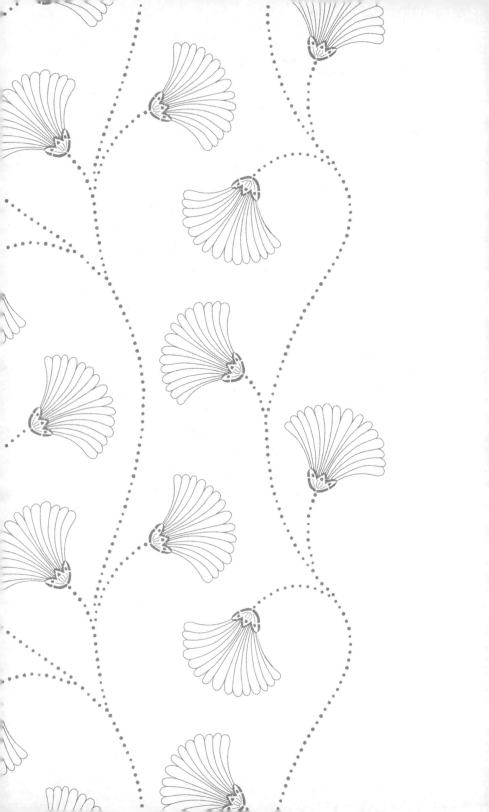

15

A Pinterest-Perfect Nursery

Pinterest's algorithm thought I would be interested in creating an accent wall in Selah's nursery using gold-dot decals.

Pinterest was right.

I deliberated over paint colors, committed to a soft shade of pink—less bubblegum and more ballet slipper—and ordered a package of the gold decals that had been found for me. I'm both an aspiring minimalist and a sucker for social-media ads.

Dan and I made plans to put the decals on the wall on a Friday night. We dragged our kitchen chairs up the stairs, grabbed a level and a pencil, and ripped open the package. It was then that I realized I hadn't given any thought to how we would get the dots onto the wall in the perfect, staggered rows I envisioned.

We jokingly call this the night our marriage almost ended.

Perhaps we were doomed from the start: Dan has the skills needed to visualize a space, calculate how to execute the vision, and measure and mark and complete the task—though he would prefer to wing it. I, on the other hand, possess an unfaltering belief that I am always right and an inner drive to achieve perfection—though I lack all practical skills when it comes to completing home projects.

As I climbed onto a chair, I tried to explain the plan I had devised moments ago, which involved creating a grid of Christmas ribbons across the wall and checking my work three different ways before placing a single dot. Dan tried to explain that his plan was to forget the dots altogether, but if I was committed to them, it would be far simpler to place a dot and then measure the distance to the next one as we went along. I heard, "Your plan is dumb, and so are these dots." He heard, "I don't trust your plan, and I'll blame you if this goes wrong, so let's do it my way."

We tried my method first, and I quickly realized Dan was right in at least one way—my plan was unnecessarily complicated. I begrudgingly consented to try his idea, which I was still convinced would lead to uneven rows. And while I hate to admit it, I actually felt frustrated when it became clear that his method was both more accurate and more efficient, torn as I was between my desire to be right and my desire to have those dots perfectly positioned.

Later that night, with half the decals on the wall, we let the sun go down on our frustration when we became too tired to see straight. It took a few days of gathering our courage before we could reenter the nursery and place the remainder of the dots.

There was also a lot of apologizing (mostly on my part) after I-told-you-so moments, mutual relief when we finished, and genuine admiration because the wall looked as lovely as Pinterest had promised it would. I moved the crib into place and felt myself exhale with relief. The nursery wasn't done, but I could cross this particular project off my to-do list.

I continued working on the room in the weeks that followed and often found myself swept away by reveries. As I stocked the dresser with diapers, I imagined tickling Selah's tummy while she lay on the changing pad. As I folded her sleepers, I pictured my hands gently guiding her arms and legs into them and snapping the buttons one by one. As I tucked blankets into a drawer, I thought about how delicious it would be to snuggle her with the crocheted creations draped over us.

Other times, these same tasks dredged up panic and indecision: I arranged her clothes only to rearrange them over and over in more practical ways, searched online for the perfect basket to hold her hair bows, and moved the diapers from one drawer to another and then back again, trying to determine the most sensible location. Looking back, I'm tempted to roll my eyes at these behaviors, but I also feel a tenderness toward the woman I was, and sometimes still am: I wanted to get it right. I wanted to create a lovely space for my child. I wanted to feel prepared.

Surely, I thought, a prepared mom would have a complete, coordinated nursery ready for her baby—even if it wouldn't stay that way for long. I knew I would eventually be too busy and tired to painstakingly fold every pair of baby pajamas, and someday an active toddler would pull the neatly organized books off the shelves. The rest of my house and the rest of my life would surely be in disarray for a while too.

There would soon be a crying infant I couldn't console, nightmares I couldn't soothe, accidents I couldn't prevent. I would face tantrums that would test me and changes I wouldn't know how to handle. I was bound to make mistakes—mistakes that would carry more weight than ever before. And though I couldn't imagine what it would actually feel like, I knew I'd be overcome with a love so instinctual, so ferocious, that it might threaten to consume me. My life would no longer be exclusively mine.

As I came face to face with this overwhelming reality, putting together the nursery offered to be my last fling with perfection. Selah's room was the one thing I could do perfectly before the chaos of life with a tiny human arrived.

I can't remember a time when I didn't have an inner drive for perfection. In school, I was the kid who hated arts-and-crafts time because I could never fold the paper perfectly in half or cut a razor-straight line. When practicing cursive, I would form a letter and then erase it, form and erase, form and erase, until my paper was smudged and marked by the holes I'd worn through it in my frustration.

As an adult, my need for perfection and order has manifested in more subtle but perhaps more damaging ways. I've attempted to conform my body into the perfect shape. I avoid taking risks or making decisions without first carefully crafting a plan. I agonize over tiny decisions such as where to eat for date night or what to wear to a party, thinking there is one perfect option available, and I am responsible for identifying it. I subconsciously believe that having all the details of a situation ordered and complete can provide a guarantee that I'll be able to handle any surprises that might come my way. And so my thinking with the nursery went something like this: *If I can make it perfect, down to the very last detail, I'll feel ready to have my world—and this room—turned upside down.*

But the thing is, I rarely get to the point where I believe I *do* have everything in order. I never achieve my elusive definitions of preparedness and perfection. My choices eat away at me as I wonder whether I've made the right decision, and I feel uncomfortable and insecure, never quite capturing the confidence and rest "perfection" had promised me.

Once the walls were painted and the dots arranged in neat rows, I began to hunt for a glider chair. These chairs are not cheap, and I hesitated to spend so much money on a single piece of furniture, but all my friends said if I was going to buy a chair for the space, it would be well worth it to invest in one that was both comfortable and built to last. "You'll be spending *hours* in that chair, often in the middle of the night," they told me. "You'll want it to be a happy, cozy place." After hours of research and reading reviews and testing them out in the store, I found one I hoped would be worth the expense.

When Dan placed the chair in the corner of the nursery, tucked between the window on one wall and the crib on the other, my inner fretting paused. I settled my growing body into the chair, propped my feet up on the matching ottoman, and closed my eyes, captivated by a daydream once again. Here I would hold my newborn baby, my arms cradling her body and supporting her head, my fingertips grazing her tiny toes. Here I would sing lullabies over her as she drifted off to sleep, my voice providing a sense of comfort and security. Here we would read bedtimes stories and snuggle close as she grew, eventually able to climb in and out of my lap on her own.

Early in the mornings when I couldn't sleep (thanks to pregnancy insomnia), I would cross the hallway to the nursery to knock a few tasks off my to-do list. The first thing I saw every time I opened the door was the cream-colored chair, and despite the swirling thoughts I had entered the room with, the sight of it slowed me down. It felt as if I were being invited to rest for one more minute, to dream about all that would take place in this room, to envision the home it would become for my little girl.

As I rocked in the chair each day, a quiet meditation before jumping into productivity, I realized my quest for a Pinterest-perfect nursery had never really been about perfection for the sake of it—something softer had simply gotten caught in the trap of perfectionism. My efforts were reflective of the deep love I already felt for my little girl and my desire to welcome her into our home and say, "You're ours! You belong here!" I wanted her nursery to be a sanctuary for both of us in the chaotic days to come, a place where we could retreat for security, familiarity, and connection.

Perfectionism is often a shortsighted attempt at connection. We want to be loved, so we strive to be as worthy of love as possible. We want to be seen as capable and dependable and unflappable, and somehow that gets translated to never making mistakes. We want to make others feel comfortable and cared for, so we hide all the clutter before guests arrive, make sure we look put together, and warn our kids to be on their best behavior.

But it doesn't work. Though we hope our perfection will facilitate connection, it's actually a hindrance to the very thing we're after. As we try harder and do more, as we overvalue productivity and perfection, we fly past the moments of connection that start from a place of rest, vulnerability, and attunement to others.

Take this gold-dot debacle as an example (a cautionary tale, even): what could have been a fun night of working as a team with my husband, talking about our hopes and dreams for our baby girl while we added a touch of whimsy to her room, devolved into a tense standoff. I wanted perfection and didn't trust anyone but myself to get us there, and so I missed the opportunity for connection.

Later, when Selah turned one, I whipped myself into a frenzy while I decorated and cleaned and cooked, doing my best to make her party just right—so much so that I hardly remember any of the details. I was so tired and overwhelmed by the time our guests arrived that I wished I could go upstairs and sleep rather than engage and enjoy.

I can recognize that in these scenarios, and in the dozens of other examples from my life, I had the best of intentions. I simply wanted to show my people how much I love them. But as it turns out, they don't measure my love in all-or-nothing terms (if it's not a perfect display, it's worthless). They feel loved through my attempt, however imperfect my efforts end up.

If you, too, struggle with perfectionism, consider this my invitation to you. Before jumping into action, whether on decorating the nursery or reading another parenting book or planning a birthday party, think about what it would look like to prioritize connection. Before trying to prove your ability or worth, take a minute to be still. Before spiraling into control and perfectionism, remember a higher purpose: to lay a foundation of beauty, peace, and security as an expression of love for your child.

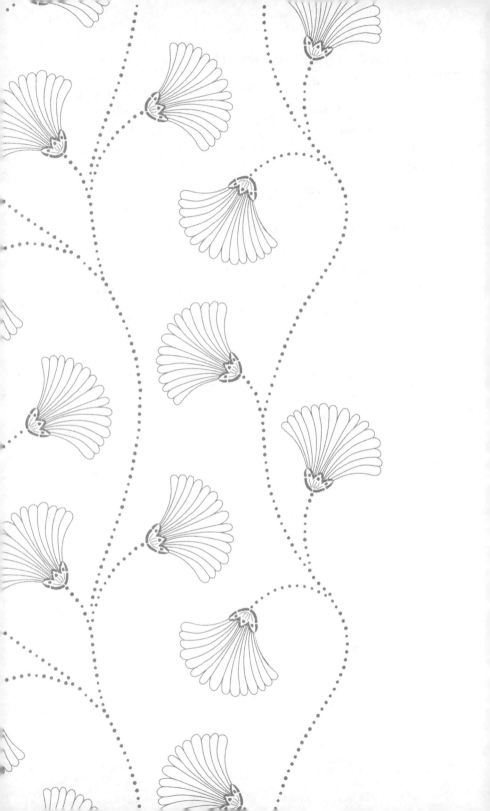

16

Working Mom

I took a job teaching first grade at a charter school outside of Gary, Indiana, when I was fresh out of college and barely twenty-two. I spent long hours in the classroom, hours filled by constant interaction with tiny humans. All day long, I had to be "on," and I was regularly on the brink of losing my mind when I couldn't get just five minutes alone. I desperately wanted to believe this was God's calling for me—yet I was drained and unhappy, anxious and frustrated, exhausted and overwhelmed.

Does this mean I'm a failure? I wondered often. *Why is this not fulfilling?* As it turned out, I wasn't a failure—I was a highly sensitive introvert doing a job that didn't fit my personality, skills, or working style. I couldn't have put it into those words at the time, but I knew something had to change.

After a few years in the classroom, I joined the staff at an educational nonprofit as an instructional and leadership coach for new teachers. I was deeply passionate about and invested in the work, and managing adults rather than working directly with students brought some relief. But like teaching, this job involved long and odd hours, instability, and near-constant interaction. I couldn't shake the feeling that it didn't fit, like shoes that were the wrong size, rubbing and pinching in all the wrong spots. Sure, those shoes carried me from point A to point B, but I was left tired and sore and a tiny bit broken.

The spring after Dan and I got married, I had to decide whether I would commit to another school year of coaching. We both agreed it wasn't the right fit for me or for the future I envisioned as a working mom. I came home each day as the worst version of myself—exhausted, crabby, and quick to snap—and that's not the me I wanted to be when I was at home with my (then-theoretical) kids. But if I wasn't going to teach or coach, what on earth would I do?

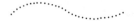

While most eight-year-olds were plotting out elaborate imaginative games, I was planning which college I would attend and what my long-term career trajectory would be. Some days I wanted to attend Juilliard and be a Broadway star. Most days I wanted to attend Harvard and be a lawyer, then a senator, and then president. I wasn't particularly interested in having children; I loved playing house with my friends and taking care of our "babies," but in real life, I was more interested in climbing the ladder than in carrying diaper bags and wiping noses.

As a member of the millennial generation, the foundational question of my life was, *What do I want to be when I grow up?* My parents asked me, their friends asked me, my teachers asked me. I grew up attending Take Our Daughters and Sons to Work Days and career days at school. I believed my primary responsibility in life was to find a profession I was passionate about, and everything else would fall into place.

I showed up at college ready to take the next step toward a distinguished career. But along the way, the college ministry I was involved with introduced me to a theology that asserted women should work only until they became mothers, and I bought in—so much so that I chose elementary education as my major to really embrace that motherly identity.

Looking back, I realize my driving motivation in life was (and still is) to do things the right way. I make sense of this enormous shift in my career trajectory by remembering that motivation. If this was supposedly the "right" way to be a woman, then I had to do it. With that, the foundational question of my life changed from *What do I want to be?* to *Who do others think I should be?*

This decision troubled the friends and family members who knew me best, but I tried to make everyone—myself included—believe this was my calling from God. It worked for a while: I found jobs that married my degree in education with my heart for social justice. But what I thought would be the epic saga of my life turned out to be a short story when I burned out just five years in.

I sat in my car one afternoon shortly after I had turned in my notice for the instructional coaching job. I had a few minutes to spare before meeting with a teacher, so I continued listening to the radio as a guest shared the impetus for her recent big life change. A friend had asked her, "If you could do anything, within reason, what would you do?" It sounds so simple, but it had been a long time since I'd thought about my career that way. I'd been stuck thinking about what I *should* do, not what I *wanted* to do.

I rested my head on the steering wheel and whispered, "God, what desires have I kept stuffed inside in all these years? Who did you create me to be?" And to myself, I asked the most vulnerable questions of all: *Who am I? What do I want?*

A single word began to bounce around my brain: *books.* I'd loved books and stories and words for as long as I could remember. Before I could read, I would scan the letters in my American Girl books as my mom read aloud to me, mumbling under my breath and repeating what she said, mesmerized by the cadence of the sentences. I knew right then that if I could do anything, within reason, I would work with books.

I began to research jobs in the publishing world and stumbled across editing. I devoured blogs detailing what it takes to break into the publishing industry and what the work is really like—of course, it's less glamorous than most people would envision. I took an online class in copyediting, began drafting writing samples, and sat for self-imposed proofreading tests. I applied for jobs, got rejected, took an unpaid internship, and waited tables to help make ends meet. And eventually, I landed a job as a copyeditor at a publishing house.

After years of denying my personality type and pretending to enjoy teaching, taking on this role felt like I was finally inching closer to who I am and who I wanted to be. My days were no longer filled with the chaos of managing thirty very young children; there was sometimes chaos to be managed on the page, but that kind of chaos didn't cling to my leg and shout my name over and over again. I was surrounded by words, books, and other like-minded people (often fellow introverts) who loved those things as well. I quickly grew accustomed to the stable hours and the fact that I could leave my work at work. When I arrived home at the end of the day, I had the energy to go to the gym and cook dinner and even start a side hustle as a blogger and freelance writer. Maybe most important of all, I had the freedom to choose rest over any of those options.

My job isn't perfect. No job or organization or institution gets it all right all the time. But for the first time in my life, I felt like I could see myself in this career, if not at this company, long term—even with a few kids at home. It seemed like I could have the best of both worlds.

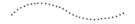

As my belly and ankles swelled in the late-summer heat, almost a year after I'd started this new job, I began to plan for my maternity leave. I created an exhaustive list of all my projects, made detailed notes about my role in each one and where it was in the process, and assigned a point person to take over should I go into labor early. Each Friday I revised the list, updating the status of each project and removing items I had finished.

I harbored some fears about how I'd be able to balance it all after a huge life change. I loved my job and felt energized by its predictability, but there was so much that was entirely unknown and unpredictable about how I would respond to motherhood, what my baby would be like, and how that would impact my work. Sheryl Sandberg says in her book *Lean In* that career paths are less like ladders and more like jungle gyms; if that's the case, then I suppose motherhood is a web of tightropes with no clear destination in sight.

There was no doubt in my mind that I wanted to return to this job. In my role as a copyeditor I had discovered my gifts and become more fully myself, which allowed me to finally be at peace with my desire not to be a stay-at-home mom. I knew and admired many women who had chosen that path and flourished in it, and I also knew it wasn't right for me, at least not right now. But for all my certainty about returning to work, there was much uncertainty about who I would be when I did. Would I still be capable and reliable? Would I feel divided? Would I eventually default to becoming a stay-at-home mom, not because I wanted to but simply because it was too hard to be a good mother and a good employee?

For every uncertain question that looped through my mind, though, there was a hopeful thought that returning to work could be exactly what I needed to help me weather the transition to motherhood. There would be immense challenges, but perhaps my job would be the very thing to keep me from losing an essential part of myself during this massive identity shift.

Maybe working will help me feel connected to my old self and remember I am Woman Brittany and not just Mommy Brittany, I told myself. *Maybe I'll long for my quiet office after a night of listening to my baby cry. Maybe my daughter will be proud of me and what I do. Maybe she'll tell her friends that her mommy works with real authors on real books. Maybe she'll see that she doesn't have to pick between a career she loves and a family she loves. Maybe she'll see in me that God can and does call women to both.*

While listening to a podcast midway through my pregnancy, I heard the host explain what working motherhood had meant for her as her family dynamic and job responsibilities had changed over the years. She said everything in life had a set of benefits and tradeoffs, and that's true in motherhood too. Staying at home has benefits and tradeoffs, as does working full time outside the home, as does any other place in between—working part time or working from home or working seasonally. We are privileged if we have the ability to choose our set of benefits and tradeoffs, and we are not locked into our decisions forever.

Around this same time, I told an experienced working mom in my department that I was certain about coming back to work but nervous about what this next phase would be like and whether I'd be able to handle it. She told me, matter-of-factly, "Give it a year. You can do anything for a year. It's long enough for the dust to settle at work and at home, and if you need to change course after that, you'll be making a clearheaded and informed decision."

Those became my mantras whenever I got swept up in all the unknowns and moving pieces of the impending changes: *I choose my benefits and tradeoffs* and *I can do anything for a year.*

All we can do is choose a scenario that seems to be the best fit for ourselves and our families and see how that decision plays out one day at a time, one season at a time, one year at a time. What works at first doesn't have to work forever. What doesn't work can be altered. We are allowed to change our minds, choose a different way, or cut a new path altogether.

In both editing and motherhood, I found what I was searching for all along: *vocation*. Not just a career, not solely a piece of my identity, not even a calling, exactly. A vocation is not any one thing: a specific calling to this job or that one, to working motherhood or stay-at-home motherhood. Any number of areas can compose our vocations— mothering, working, caregiving, volunteering, creative pursuits, hobbies, relationships, commitments. When one area ebbs, another might flow; sometimes we may need to drop one or more pieces.

The beauty of vocation is that dropping or adding a piece doesn't fundamentally change who we are. But if we engage in the process thoughtfully, honestly, and tenaciously, perhaps we will draw closer to who we've always been.

And whether or not the full picture of our vocation is all we want it to be (really, when is it ever?), God is with us in our good work. God gives us the freedom to play with the questions *Who am I?* and *What do I want?* And God is honored when we discover new and exciting answers that inch us closer to who we were created to be.

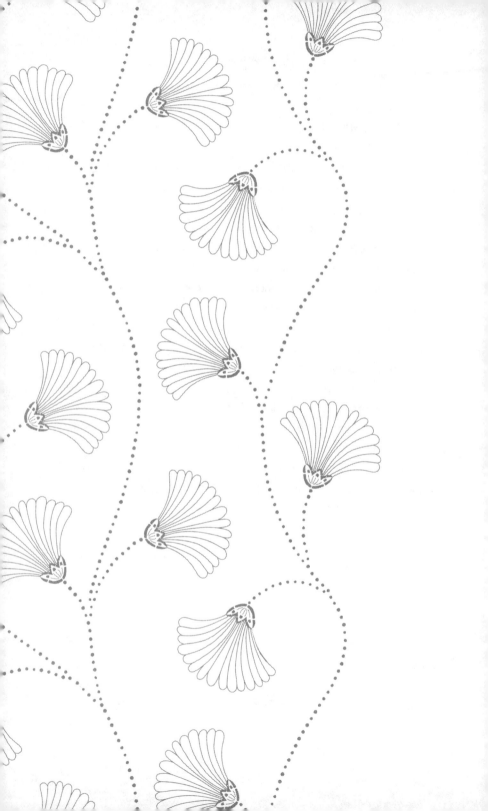

17

Making Space

My vision started to swim as I debated whether to delete a comma. The copyediting project I was working on had been my biggest challenge yet in this still-new job: there were lots of obscure facts to check, tricky endnotes to format, and awkward sentences to smooth out. More than a few times that day, I'd wanted to pull out my hair. My abilities were stretched past their maximum, and I felt like an impostor—or, at the very least, an amateur.

I still loved my job, but all jobs have their stressful periods, and this one was compounded by the strain of a major life transition and the hormones that were messing with my ability to cope.

Shortly before it was time to head home, a coworker from another department stopped by my desk to share a piece of feedback. I don't remember exactly what the situation was, but I know it was something small—I'd made a communication error or forgotten some step in a process. That day, though, it wouldn't have mattered much if my mistake had been minuscule or colossal in scale; I would have reacted the same way.

As my coworker walked away from my desk, I tried to stifle the tears pooling in my eyes and push down the achy knot building in my throat. I was embarrassed that I'd made a mistake, of course, because I want to be seen as competent and reliable. When I miss the mark, I'm incredibly hard on myself. But that day, my reaction wasn't only about my own embarrassment or what my coworker might have thought of me. The pressure behind my stress valve had been building and building for weeks, and this moment had simply forced it open.

The baby's room was nowhere near done. I was having trouble sleeping and was completely exhausted. Family events and birthday parties and one-on-one commitments punctuated nearly every week-end until my due date, which is one of the most overwhelming scenarios I can imagine as an introvert. I was still on a steep learning curve at my new job, and while some days I was proud of how much progress I'd made in less than a year, other days I felt inadequate. My nerves were stretched tight and felt about as brittle as a thin, glassy sheet of ice, shat-tered by what normally would have been a benign interaction.

As I sat at my desk crying, finally releasing the toxic sludge of all my pent-up emotions, my mind raced ten steps ahead. *If I'm struggling to keep up with my to-do list now,* I thought to myself, *how on earth will I keep up once there's a baby to care for? Something will have to give, but what?*

Over dinner that night, I told Dan about my encounter with my coworker and spilled even more word vomit about the other stressors weighing on me.

"At this rate, I feel like we'll be going, going, going until the very moment Selah is born, and I don't want to be," I lamented over my bowl of stir-fry, which had gone cold during my monologue.

Dan promised we would devote all of Sunday to working on the nursery together, and he encouraged me to completely clear at least two upcoming weekends, even if it meant canceling on people I cared about. I agreed with him and was grateful to have someone giving me the permission I couldn't give myself, but I also felt as though canceling some plans wouldn't be enough. I could wipe my calendar clean for the entire third trimester, but if I didn't intentionally connect with my body and my baby and my soul, it would all be a waste, and I'd simply find other ways to fill the time: with Netflix and novels and hours of second-guessing every nursery-related decision.

What I was truly craving was *space*: not just space on the calendar to get things done but space to rest, to process, and to open my eyes to the transformation happening inside me. I wanted to enjoy every minute I had left of being pregnant, every gradual physical change, every squirmy baby kick. In the midst of the busyness and the to-dos that come along with preparing for a baby, it had started to feel like pregnancy was happening *to* me while I wasn't paying attention. I didn't want to wake up one day and realize there was a newborn baby in my arms—I wanted to be a conscious part of bringing her into the world, starting now.

I did take Dan's advice and canceled some plans, and then I took it a step further by vowing to say no to every other incoming invitation for the time being. Part of me was still afraid that by saying no—something I was not used to doing—I would alienate the people I loved. I genuinely cared about attending my cousin's wedding shower, I wanted to catch up with the coworker who had invited me to lunch, and I knew a dear friendship would benefit from a good, long chat over a cup of coffee. But if it was all at the expense of my mental health, would any of that be worth it?

Clearing space in my calendar cleared space in my mind too—instead of charging ahead, I had time to listen to and heed what my body was telling me. I took naps, went for quiet walks, and watched Selah move beneath my skin just for the pleasure of it. I journaled about what I was feeling, releasing all the uncertainty onto the page instead of letting it build up inside like a pressure cooker. And when there was less stress in my body, I found myself sleeping longer and less fitfully.

Every time I said, "I'm sorry, but I can't," I felt a little light flicker on inside me, a little piece of my "no" muscle grow stronger. I still had no idea how I would fit a baby into my life, but the more nos I said and the more space I created, the more it seemed possible. And the more I filled the resulting space with activities that helped me connect to the present, the more I felt like an active participant in what was happening to my body and soul.

Perhaps making space for a baby isn't about taking a few things off our to-do lists and expecting motherhood to slide neatly into the gaps. Instead, I think we need to be willing to obliterate our to-do lists—and our expectations too—carefully choosing what to allow back in rather than choosing what to let go of in the first place.

One thing we don't need to allow back into our lives is the pressure to do everything, and do it well. We must learn to make hard decisions to preserve our mental health and, therefore, the health of our families. We have to decide what is and isn't worth doing and then learn to say no to the latter. We have to get comfortable with saying no now so we'll be strong enough to say far more important nos when our babies arrive: no to housekeeping, no to the pressure to fit into our prebaby jeans, no to the need to appear Instagram ready at all times, no to going out when we need to stay in and snuggle our babies. No to the kind of mom that culture wants us to be and no to the brand of motherhood we see on social media: women who are perfectly made up while they push out their squeaky-clean babies, who jump back into the breakneck pace of regular life just days after giving birth.

By saying these all-important nos, we free ourselves to say yes to our own kind of motherhood: one that starts, first, with a healthy and secure mother. In a way, it seems counterintuitive and selfish. After all, aren't mothers supposed to sacrifice themselves for the sake of their babies, to be inexhaustibly self-giving? But in the case of pregnancy, caring for ourselves is exactly the same as caring for our children.

And maybe that doesn't end when our children no longer share our bodies. Caring for ourselves makes us healthier moms, ready to model health to our kids and love them from a place of fullness.

Let's say no to excessive scheduling and yes to margin.

Let's say no to cultural pressure and impossible standards and yes to forging our own paths.

Let's say no to having it all figured out and a resounding yes to letting ourselves off the hook.

Let's say no to depletion and yes to meeting our needs.

Third Trimester

Anticipating Change and Welcoming Wonder

18

Dormancy

Dan's family has a waterfront cottage on the Chain of Lakes up near the Illinois-Wisconsin border. Whenever I talk about spending time there, I feel the need to qualify it. The one-bedroom cabin was built in 1927, and Dan's dad remodeled the entire thing by himself in the 1970s. The whole cottage is monochromatic: the cedar siding is brown; the floors are brown-and-cream linoleum; the kitchen has dark-brown cabinets and tan countertops; the hand-me-down couches are an orangey-brown leather, the surfaces cracked and faded with age.

It's not fancy, but you can feel the love and nostalgia in the walls, and being at the cottage is what makes summer feel like summer. We rarely run the air conditioning, opting instead to let the breeze from the lake cool the house. There's always a spread of food on the counters: bowls of freshly cut watermelon, open bags of popcorn to grab by the handful, a plastic container filled with the almond-meal chocolate chip cookies I have come to associate with Dan's mom.

Dan and I spent many weekends at the cottage the summer before the baby was due. I sat in the sun and read novel after novel, and we feasted on charcoal-grilled burgers and kettle-cooked chips and corn on the cob slathered in butter. We went out for boat rides in the heat of the day and as the sun was setting, and I would drape a lavender crocheted blanket over my legs and marvel at the sherbet skies hovering above the water. Dan's dad drove the boat slowly when I was on board—maybe slower than necessary—insistent on protecting me and his growing grandbaby.

The cottage was one of the few places where I didn't feel pressure to be productive, where I felt a rare freedom to be spontaneous by sneaking in one last boat ride or running over to Dairy Queen for Blizzards. In the sunshine of summer, my November due date seemed far off, with plenty of time left for me to figure everything out: how I would get through childbirth, how I would breastfeed and care for an infant and survive on little sleep, how I would rise to the occasion of being someone else's mother, how I would handle the enormity of being responsible for another person's health and growth and well-being.

As much as I enjoyed my prebaby summer, however, fall has long been my favorite season. In the Midwest, winter is brutally cold, and summer is brutally humid. Spring doesn't offer much relief from the bitterness of winter, with its unrelenting cloudiness and its cold, pelting rain. But fall: it is both painfully short and gloriously pleasant.

Everything glitters in the fall. The sky is shockingly blue, dotted with white clouds reminiscent of the iconic wallpaper from *Toy Story*. The trees are ablaze with jewel tones, turning from summer's emerald to gold and ruby and citrine. I stand ready to break out my sweaters at the first sign of an autumn breeze and to gather with friends for a backyard bonfire.

As a child, I was always eager for the coming of fall, the smell of freshly sharpened pencils and new books rising like incense to mark the beginning of a new school year. Even as an adult, the onset of autumn evokes the sense of being on the edge of something new and exciting and slightly scary.

As we left the lake for the last time that year, the leaves were already beginning their metamorphosis. That same mix of anticipation and apprehension was building inside me. With one hand on my belly and the other trailing outside my open window, I thought about all the change that was coming as we ushered in a new season.

Throughout my pregnancy, I'd been thinking of fall as Baby Time, when time would start to slip away along with the extra hours of daylight. I had a vague idea of what was coming, but in the same optimistic way a kid knows what's coming in adulthood: eating ice cream for breakfast just because you can, working at a "real" job that requires a professional wardrobe, getting coffee with friends on the weekends.

As a mom-to-be standing a safe distance from her due date, I could imagine a similar caricature of all the sweet parts of life with a newborn: squishy snuggles and first smiles and all the gurgles and coos to come. The closer I got to November, however, the more reality set in. Like a kaleidoscope shifting to reveal a new pattern, the change in the seasons added some depth and clarity to what I imagined the baby days would hold: a broken body, leaky breasts, precious little sleep, inconsolable crying (mine and the baby's), endless poopy diapers.

Our car picked up speed on a stretch of road that sees little traffic, the foliage and colors blurring together in my peripheral vision, out of focus and out of reach. *Will I even recognize myself in this next season?* I wondered. *Amid the chaos, will I be able hear the voices that matter— my own voice, my maternal instinct, God?*

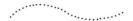

In nature, the autumn months function as a time of preparation. Where the summer sun yields rapid growth, the dropping temperatures of fall prompt harvest: a time to collect the abundance of summer before the first frost sets in and to store up what is needed to survive winter. Plants release their seeds to be carried off by the wind, trusting in the promise of dormancy and of new growth when creation awakens from its sleeping state.

As the baby grew, so did my sense of needing to prepare, to nest, to make things feel ready and complete. The seasons would soon turn again, and I would begin my own stretch of dormancy, performing only the basic functions needed for survival. In preparation, I gathered ingredients and stored away freezer meals; I checked items off my to-do list; I began to wrap up tasks at work.

The sun continued to rise later and set earlier, and as the days grew shorter I began to draw inward. I couldn't help it: it was like a biological impulse to go dormant. I continued to say no to invitations and clear off my autumn schedule. I declined new writing projects and set up an email autoresponse. At times it felt like my creative stream had run dry entirely, but I see now that it had been redirected to the work of growing my daughter.

One weekend, while attending a blogging conference I'd been looking forward to for months, I was overcome by a visceral feeling of homesickness. It made no sense to me: I love to travel, and I especially love attending workshops and conferences because they allow me to be a student again. People I had known only online were now with me in person, sharing stories and eating meals together. It should have been a dream come true.

But this wave of homesickness was so profound that I could not escape it; I *needed* to be in a place where I was fully known and entirely comfortable. I cried in my room the second night there, overwhelmed and confused by the power of this sensation. Even though there was only one day and one night left in my trip, I packed my bags and drove home the next morning.

I pulled into my driveway around noon, and Dan came outside to meet me and haul my suitcase inside. As I stepped over the threshold to our house, I was enveloped by a relief so deep and instant that I knew I'd made the right choice for my mental health. Within minutes, I had changed into sweatpants and collapsed onto the couch. Our dog, Riley, nestled herself next to me, her head resting on my belly. We stayed there for hours while I read and absentmindedly scratched her ears, both of us saturated with peace.

In my newfound dormancy, I clung to these moments of calm and introspection, knowing they were transitory and fleeting. The rocking chair in my daughter's nursery became a safe place where I could let myself feel my competing emotions. I rocked forward and back, moving toward the end of my pregnancy and anticipating a new beginning as a mother—as a version of myself I had never been before, a version I hoped I would recognize and like and be proud of.

The world around me kept moving, inching toward autumn and then winter. The tension between the outer movement and my inward stillness reminded me that every year, the seasons come and go, always in the same order. We can savor the present, but we can't camp out in one part of the year and circumvent change.

As we give ourselves to these rhythms, we learn to anticipate the goodness of each season, even the ones that feel desolate and lonely. The only way to the regeneration of spring and the fruit of summer is through death in fall and dormancy in winter.

Likewise, the only way to our new identities as moms is through a willingness to let go of pieces of ourselves, the way a tree releases its leaves, trusting that something both new and familiar will take their place.

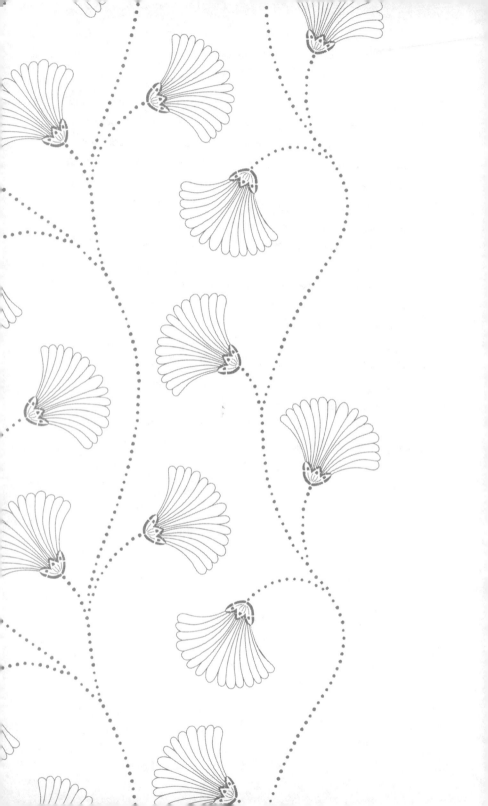

19

Movement

I sat on the couch one Saturday morning, reading a novel and relishing one of my two allotted cups of coffee for the day, when Selah's feet began to swish against and then knead the top of my stomach. I quickly shifted the mug off my belly shelf, her movements wild enough to slosh the coffee onto my hand.

I placed my book on the couch, grabbed my phone, and opened the camera app to video her kicks. I knew someday I would want to look back on this moment, to relive the kicks that would soon exist only in my memory, to be drawn back into the sweetness of the time when my wiggly daughter made her home in my body.

As I savored each of Selah's movements, she reminded me to savor other tiny wonders as well: the morning sunlight streaking through the windows of my living room, falling asleep on the couch on a Sunday afternoon, leaving the windows open on those first cool nights of autumn, the scent of fresh sheets as I climbed into bed.

Time seemed to be moving faster every day—if my life were a low-budget made-for-TV movie, the calendar pages would be tearing off and blowing away with an unexplained gust of wind. But each of Selah's movements felt like an invitation to be immersed in the present moment, to slow down my perception of time, even if I couldn't change its actual pace.

The first time I felt my daughter move was nothing like I had seen it portrayed on TV. One of my favorite misrepresentations of this phenomenon is from *Friends*: in the middle of an impromptu game of spin the bottle, Phoebe shouts, "Oh my God, the baby just kicked!" The whole gang rushes over to feel her belly, derailing Rachel's plan to kiss her crush.

For me, it happened far more gradually and privately. At first I wasn't even sure if the baby was moving or if I was just feeling gas bubbles from my nightly LaCroix. There would be a tiny swish of movement along my abdominal wall, and then it was gone, sometimes for days at a time, leaving me to wonder whether I'd really felt anything at all. Over time, Selah's movements become more pronounced but not quite identifiable: some limb bumping up against me, the brush of a hand or a foot. It was many weeks later before Dan could feel her moving from the outside, and even longer before the movement was visible.

In the middle of the third trimester I reached the "alien belly" stage, where the baby's kicks and rolls would send ripples of movement across the surface of my stretched stomach. Her feet were up near the top of my belly, her legs tucked slightly, and every time she stretched it felt like there was a rolling massage chair inside me. Her head and hands were positioned down near my pelvis and her butt right at my belly button, and sometimes she would move all at once, stretching her arms and pushing her butt up and out, which I pictured as an in utero version of downward dog.

Other movements left me puzzled, and I wondered whether I would recognize them once she was outside the womb, thinking, *Oh, that's what you were doing in there!* In the final weeks of pregnancy my belly became so tight and her movements so forceful that I couldn't believe her little feet weren't bursting right through the amniotic sac.

Before pregnancy, I had not felt particularly connected to my body. It's not even that I felt *disconnected* from it but rather that I didn't realize there was a connection to be made. I lived in my head, thinking of my body as a tool with which I could execute my thoughts and desires, an object I could command and subdue, rather than a living thing that is valuable in its own right.

But now there was another person living inside my body, someone who was growing and developing without much intervention from me. I provided the nutrients and a safe space in which she could thrive, but I was not causing her fingers to grow longer or her eyelashes to sprout; I did not tell her heart to start beating or remind her to practice sucking her thumb and swallowing amniotic fluid. Every tiny flutter and swift kick felt like an expression of her will, a reminder that I was both separate from and deeply connected to her through my body, through the bone and blood and tissue that formed each of us.

Every time my belly moved, free of my will, it was as if light was cracking over the horizon at dawn, spilling out bit by bit. I was amazed at what my body could do—build an entire human from a single egg and a single sperm—but I was even more amazed by how much this process grounded me in my own physicality. The distinction between body and soul now felt arbitrary: I wasn't just a soul residing in a body. My body was a *home*. And that meant my body was good, safe, something to be trusted.

Almost involuntarily, whenever the baby started to kick, I stopped whatever I was doing to place a hand on my belly: first thing in the morning or last thing at night, in the middle of my workday or while watching Netflix with Dan. Sometimes I would push gently on my stomach to see whether she would kick back, or I'd eat a piece of chocolate if I hadn't felt her move in a while, hoping the sugar would get her going. The sensation of her movement never became old or boring—if anything, I grew more surprised at her increasing strength and astonished at the ability of my abdomen to withstand her force.

As she pushed against my stomach, I wondered about her motivations: Was she feeling cramped and needing more space? Was she trying to break free? Was she entertaining herself? Was she trying to get my attention? She knew nothing of life outside the womb, of course, but her movements felt both playful and purposeful—she was building strength in her legs and practicing using her arms. I pictured her blinking her newly formed eyelids and blowing bubbles, motions I had seen on ultrasounds. Her playfulness connected me to the joy of pregnancy rather than the fear that often dominated my experience.

With every kick, I became more attuned to her body, her desires, her needs, her will. She wasn't kicking because she actually needed me, but eventually she would do other things to get my attention: she would cry, coo, and root at my breast in an effort to make herself heard and get her needs met.

When our babies are born, it can seem like overnight a switch has flipped and we are, for the first time, completely attuned to another person's body. We watch for the precious rise and fall of their chests, for signs of sleepiness or hunger or stress. When we see these signs, we swoop in to meet those very needs, our physical bodies mingling, once again, with our babies': scooping our little ones into our arms, using our hands to warm up a bottle or unhook our bras so they can eat, placing them on our bare chests for skin-to-skin bonding. We spend hours upon hours in those early months rocking and shushing and baby-wearing and snuggling.

There's a phenomenon I've heard about in mothers, and it was true for me after Selah was born: we can't sleep as deeply or restfully as we used to because we are listening for the needs of our babies. Especially in those early months when Selah was in a bassinet right next to my bed, I awoke to every little grunt and sniffle, sometimes even to imagined cries. I believe this attunement—our bodies listening for the bodies of our babies—is mother's intuition.

People told me throughout pregnancy that I would just *know* what my baby needed because of mother's intuition. At the time, I was skeptical of this idea, but now, having birthed and cared for two babies, I see that it's real. However, I don't think it's a magical force that gets activated as soon as we give birth. In the first weeks of new motherhood, I thought mother's intuition had skipped over me entirely, as I had no frame of reference for what was normal and when to be worried. *Is she breathing? Is she getting enough to eat? Why isn't this getting easier?*

Rather, I think mother's intuition is a skill that becomes embedded into our bodies moment by moment as we watch for signs of our babies: the pink test line, the growing curve of a belly, the first swish of movement, the breaking of water, the crowning of a head. (Or perhaps as we fill out adoption paperwork and wait with bated breath for a phone call.) This skill doesn't reach its full potential the moment our children are born but continues to grow alongside them. Each little moment of tuning our attention to the body of another builds the connection between mother and child, enabling a seemingly primal knowledge of what our babies need and deepening our confidence and identity as moms.

The word *intuition* has always felt a little woo-woo to me— hyperspiritual, intangible, maybe even fantastical. But as I felt my daughter's body move within mine, I came to see that intuition is deeply physical.

We were born with an innate understanding of our needs, and we had no problem asking someone to meet those needs. As babies, we cried for milk or for a reassuring snuggle. As toddlers, we expressed our anger freely through tantrums. We fell asleep when we were tired, asked for food when we were hungry, pushed away our plates when we were satisfied. It wasn't even a matter of listening to our bodies and then acting on what we heard. It was seamless— a normal and natural expression.

As we grew, many of us we were taught, implicitly or explicitly, to stifle our needs and subdue our desires, and this left us disconnected from our bodies, and thus from our intuitive sense of what we need. We stopped listening to our intuition, and eventually we could no longer recognize its voice.

May we take a lesson from our babies, as we watch them move and express their wills before they are even born, and as we learn along with them through each cry and giggle, each whimper and hiccup. As our mother's intuition develops, let's allow our own intuition to blossom alongside it. When our stomachs rumble even though we ate less than an hour ago, let's listen to our hunger and go grab a snack. When we feel our eyelids getting heavy in the middle of the day, let's heed that sleepy cue and let them close. When the stretchy panels of our maternity pants start to feel tight and constricting instead of gentle and supportive, let's buy bigger pants and give our changing bodies room to breathe.

Each time we listen to ourselves and take action, no matter how insignificant it seems, we rebuild the connection that was severed and learn to see our bodies as good and trustworthy and deserving of care.

20

Baby Showers

Everyone else in the cabin was sleeping as I tiptoed to the kitchen to make coffee and watch the sun rise over the mountains. Dan and I were on an extended weekend vacation with my college friends and their families, and we'd rented a log cabin near Colorado Springs.

I rounded the corner to the kitchen, rubbing my tired eyes and feeling out of sorts from the altitude and time change. A glimmer of pink caught my attention; in my quest for coffee, I'd almost missed it. Each place at the massive dining table was set with gold chargers and pink paper plates, and baby bottles stood in for glasses. Pink streamers were twisted through the antler chandelier above. A framed print that read "Congratulations, Brittany and Dan!" sat in the middle of the table, along with half a dozen gifts.

Tears filled my eyes as I wondered at the logistics and careful planning that had led to this moment: *Everyone must have sent secret texts to plan for this! How did they make room in their suitcases to pack all these gifts and decorations? And I was with them last night . . . so when did they set everything up?*

As my friends woke up one by one, I hugged them tightly and whispered my thank-yous, overwhelmed by their thoughtfulness.

We dined on French toast and bacon, toasted with our juice-filled bottles, and took dozens of pictures of the festivities. I had no idea how I would get the gifts back to Illinois—I'm a chronic overpacker, and I was already testing the strength of my suitcase's zipper—but I counted myself lucky to have such a problem.

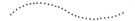

I confess that until that moment in Colorado, I had always been a bit of a baby-shower hater. It was partly because of my introversion: I don't enjoy small talk, forced merriment, or cheesy party games. I also don't like chicken salad, which often seems to be the food of choice at these events.

But the bigger reason for my aversion was that I didn't *understand* baby showers. I had attended plenty of them for my friends and always assumed they were covers for getting lots of baby gifts. In exchange for gifts, the hosts provide food and give out favors and do their best make it feel festive.

I say this without much antipathy—I've happily provided gifts for my friends' showers, because babies need a lot of stuff, and their stuff is absurdly expensive. It's what I interpreted as the false premise that bothered me. Couldn't we all admit that no one wants to eat baby food while blindfolded or mark off bingo squares filled with baby items? Couldn't we all acknowledge that we'd rather mail a gift and be spared the communal pressure to be jovial?

Besides, getting married and having babies are not the only big transitions in life. They are important milestones, of course, and they deserve to be celebrated. But it seems like we should also have showers for young adults who are moving out on their own for the first time. We should shower and equip and celebrate people when they start a new job or move across the country to chase a dream.

Since I didn't especially enjoy baby showers, I felt uncomfortable with the idea of people hosting one on my behalf. It was an undeniable privilege to have friends in my life who wanted to organize a celebration for me—not to mention that people wanted to "shower" me and this new baby with gifts to make the transition easier. But knowing how I felt about baby showers personally, I suspected others might feel the same way.

I could easily recall the pain of attending wedding and baby showers when I was so far away from those seasons myself. I would plaster a sweet smile on my face and play the games and *oooh* and *ahhh* at all the right moments, but inside a little piece of me would be shriveling, wondering, *Will I ever get married? Will I ever have children? And if I do, will anyone care?*

I hated the idea that my baby shower could cause someone else pain and that I might never know about the tears that fell when a friend opened the invitation, wishing it were her turn. I couldn't stand the thought that watching me open gifts might open a wound for someone else, that a dear friend might go home wondering whether she would ever have a chance to be celebrated in this way.

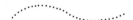

The mastermind behind my Colorado baby shower was my friend Rachel. She organized the whole thing, asked everyone to pack gifts, bought decorations, and made sure they were covertly contained in a separate suitcase. And when her husband left that suitcase at their home in Denver, she made him to drive all the way back to get it.

At the time, Rachel was also two years down the road of infertility.

That morning as I looked around the table at each of my friends, I saw genuine joy on their faces. Even Rachel, who wears her emotions on her sleeve and doesn't ever attempt to hide her pain, seemed happy to be there. No one had forced her to plan and host a celebration for me; she had done it because she loved me, because she knew I was in the midst of a personal upheaval and she wanted to walk me through it.

Rachel insisted I open gifts before eating breakfast. Her excitement was palpable, radiating through her fingertips as she handed me each package, audible in her squeals of delight over the contents. When I opened the gift from Erin—a beautiful blush-pink wrap carrier and a knitted baby sweater in the same color—I felt prepared. When I opened the gift from Eileen—a set of rhyming books about animals—I felt anticipation. And when I opened a gift from Rachel— a hand-painted pink globe with gold lettering that read "You are our greatest adventure"—I felt extravagantly loved.

I had mentioned to her once in a group text that I'd found a globe like this one on Etsy. I had designed the baby's room with the globe as my inspiration but then decided not to buy it because it cost ninety dollars and was purely decorative. Rachel immediately asked one of her craftiest friends to reproduce it for me. This gift was not a practical piece of baby gear, and it didn't bring me any closer to being prepared for the reality of life with a baby. But it made me feel seen and known and deeply loved as I was experiencing a transition we both desperately wished she were experiencing as well.

Perhaps the reason that particular brunch flipped my perception of baby showers on its head was because it didn't ignore the reality of anyone else's pain; instead, it took place amid the pain and joy we had already shared with one another that weekend. As the girls and I had planned this trip, we envisioned hiking and sightseeing and being outdoors in the Colorado sunshine as much as possible. We did some of that, but mostly we fell into a more familiar pattern. We lay around on the couches with hordes of snacks, updated everyone on the happy parts of our lives, lamented over our heartaches, and asked for help and prayer and guidance.

These women had known me since I was eighteen, and over the course of our decade-long friendship, we had experienced intense highs and lows, walked one another through the pain of breakups and rejection letters, cheered one another on as we started businesses and new jobs. We'd danced at one another's weddings and cried at airports when we had to say goodbye.

And as we sat around the table toasting with our baby bottles full of apple juice, I knew they saw *me*: not just the baby I was growing but the woman I had been, the woman I was right at that moment, and the woman I was becoming as I approached motherhood. It felt less like they were celebrating the fact that I'd accomplished the act of repro-duction and more like they were commissioning me, sending me into this new role fueled by love and prepared by my community.

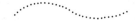

Not every baby shower captures this sense of communal commission-ing in exactly the same way, but I've seen glimpses of it. At a shower for a coworker, the hosts asked us to bring our gifts unwrapped to minimize pain for guests and awkwardness for the mom-to-be. One shower actually happened a few weeks after a friend's second baby was born, and all the guests brought a box of her preferred brand of diapers and a meal for her freezer. Another friend was encouraged to create a registry for her fourth baby, a foster son, because his needs were so unique and extensive. And one more friend used her registry to help fund safe birthing experiences for mothers in Nairobi.

Remembering each of these moments fills me with hope that as a culture, we're circling closer and closer to the heart of what it means to celebrate transitional moments well. Perhaps we're starting to realize baby showers aren't just about adorable onesies or much-needed baby gear, party favors or pink-frosted cupcakes.

Being the recipient of a baby shower can help you to identify your village—and make it far easier to accept help from those same people when you're deep in the weeds of newborn life. Maybe not everyone you party with will be part of your main support system. That's okay. There are countless voices out there offering parenting advice: the well-meaning older women who remind us to savor each moment; the jaded moms who share their birth horror stories over baby-shower finger foods; the best-selling books that offer contradictory sleep methods, each swearing to be the only way you won't be stuck rocking your child to sleep when he or she goes off to college.

But if you incline your ear, I'm guessing one or two voices will rise above the din. Not because they are the loudest but because they are familiar and trustworthy. Make them your go-to people when the noise gets overwhelming, when you need someone not just to answer your questions but to see the mom *behind* the questions—the one who is feeling lonely or angry or disillusioned or depressed.

If it takes a village to raise a child, perhaps showing up to a new mom's baby shower says, "I'm with you. I'm part of *your* village." Not only on this one Sunday afternoon but in the middle of the night when she texts a frantic question, on her first day home from the hospital when she needs a pizza delivered, on a random Wednesday when she's drowning in diapers and desperate for adult interaction.

In the moments when she's not sure she's cut out for this mother-hood thing, we show her she is and we're here to help. In the moments when she feels more isolated than ever, we remind her she is not alone. In the moments when we are both feeling pain, we can toast with apple juice in our kids' sippy cups and believe there are better days ahead.

21

Partners Becoming Parents

The rain came down thick, drowning out all other noise as the windshield wipers tried feverishly to keep up. In front of our car was a long string of blurred taillights, with no indication of what was causing the holdup. It could have been an accident blocking the road, or perhaps construction, or maybe regular Friday-night traffic made worse by the weather. Whatever the cause, it took twenty minutes to go the final mile, and I was getting hangrier with every passing minute.

When Dan and I finally arrived at the restaurant for our date, we settled into a booth, removed our wet coats, and shook off the frustration along with droplets of water. Despite how the night had started, I was grateful for the chance to finally connect with Dan after a long week, and I wondered whether this would be our last date night before the baby arrived. I took a deep breath, opened my mouth to start the conversation, and . . . nothing came out. I couldn't think of a single thing to say that wasn't related to the baby.

We had countless long, rich conversations before I got pregnant, I thought. *Surely there's something we can talk about that doesn't center around impending parenthood.*

I fidgeted with the wrapper of my straw, folding it again and again until it sprang out of my fingers.

Still no words came to mind besides, *Hey, the baby is coming soon! Do you feel ready?*

Earlier in my pregnancy I'd made an unspoken commitment to myself to try to keep the baby talk out of our date nights. I had heard of couples who tried not to talk about their kids while they were out on dates and instead discussed only things that reconnected them as people, not as parents. I thought it was worth implementing during pregnancy too.

Having made good on my promise to this point, I now wondered, *How did we get here?*

And then: *If there's nothing to talk about now, what will it be like when the baby actually arrives, or when we have multiple kids? Are we already growing too far apart?*

It's possible I was hyperaware of this dynamic in a way that wasn't healthy or helpful. My parents divorced as they were approaching the empty-nest phase, and my mom talked often about how she hoped I would do things differently in my marriage.

My mom and dad had devoted the best of their time, energy, and love into us kids and into our family unit as a whole, without ever really investing in their marriage. Looking back, I can remember my parents going on only a handful of dates when I was growing up, usually to obligatory events such as weddings and parties. They never traveled just the two of them, and anytime I saw them show each other physical affection, it felt jarring and uncomfortable to witness because it was so infrequent.

My mom never said any of this to blame their divorce on us kids; in fact, she was careful to make it clear that her and my dad's choices had led them to that point. She shared only because she wanted to prevent me from making the same mistakes.

I'd heard similar sermons preached in church and received the same premarital advice from well-meaning friends who were in the thick of parenting: "Always put your marriage first. Your kids should always come second."

In a more nuanced take, one friend told me the most intense seasons of parenting would make up only a fraction of my married life. Just as moms can become so consumed by motherhood that they don't cultivate their own hobbies and passions—and then, by the time they send their kids off into the world, they've forgotten who they are—the same can happen with marriage. We become strangers to ourselves, and our spouses become strangers to us, when we focus solely on our kids.

Though this moment in the restaurant should have seemed benign—it was a Friday night, we were both exhausted, and it had been a long and frustrating journey to get to the restaurant—instead I saw it as a crack in our partnership that would only grow larger, destabilizing our bond before we'd had much of a chance to build it up.

Dan and I had known each other for only four years, and our marriage was a young two years old. The age of a toddler. In those two short years, we had lived together for the first time, moved twice, and both gone through major career changes. I found myself wondering whether we'd done it all wrong: Was it too much change too fast? Should we have waited longer to have kids? Had we had enough time to build the "foundation" everyone talks about? Should we have gone to counseling? Should we have gone on more dates? Should we have traveled more? Should we have prayed together more, read the Bible together more, read more than a few pages of a marriage book before abandoning it? Should we have done more to protect *us*?

I rarely felt guilty for not doing the things I assumed "good" Christian couples do, like reading the Bible together every morning or praying together every night. But now my heart started to beat faster as I worried that these were the magic formulas for keeping our relationship strong, and we had ignored them. I wanted to be certain we had stored up enough connection and shared memories to ensure our marriage could weather this huge change. I wanted a guarantee that we would come out stronger somehow. I wanted assurance that we would not end up like my parents.

Countless blog posts and books have been devoted to the subject of how to prepare your marriage for a baby. But much like we can never be fully prepared personally, I don't think our marriages are ever fully ready for this kind of transition. Are there more or less ideal times to expand the family? Sure. But maybe we have less control than we think. A pregnancy might announce itself at what seems like the right time, but there's a lot that can happen in the space of nine months to make it no longer the perfect time: a layoff, the death of a loved one, the loss of financial stability.

And even if all goes smoothly for the marriage during pregnancy, I'm not convinced we can "store up" connection in vast enough quantities to ration it out in the disconnected moments of early parenting. Relationships don't work that way: they take regular, ongoing connection; surges won't protect against dry spells.

This doesn't mean we're doomed when dry spells do hit— it just means it's okay if we haven't built a vast relationship reservoir to draw from. Even in a dry spell—of emotional or physical or spiritual disconnection—we can do the most basic thing of turning toward each other.

I don't remember what Dan and I ended up talking about during dinner, but I do remember coming home still craving connection after my craving for pizza had been satisfied. We used to end our days sitting side by side in our oversized chair, watching Netflix, and snuggling. But as I got further along in pregnancy, it became increasingly uncomfortable for me to sit there, and so I usually sat across the room on the couch, my back and neck propped up with pillows.

Before Dan settled into the chair that night, I asked him to come sit with me for a few minutes. As much as my achy body would allow, I leaned into him, my head on his shoulder, my arms encircling his waist. He placed a hand on my knee, and I breathed in the scent of his skin, which always floods my body with a warm stillness and pushes out the stress. When was the last time we had shared a moment like this? I couldn't remember. But it felt like this minuscule moment held the answer I was looking for.

Lingering with Dan on the couch felt like a meditation of sorts, drawing my attention to the person of my husband and shutting out everything else that vied for my attention. Those few minutes filled me up in a place I hadn't realized was depleted, and I wondered if perhaps the marriage advice I'd received wasn't wrong, exactly, but misguided. Reading the Bible or praying together isn't the secret to a strong and healthy relationship. Rather, it's the tiny moments of connection those habits foster—the daily practice of turning toward each other and toward a common value—that fortifies our partnerships bit by bit.

As we prepare to welcome children into our families, the dynamics will necessarily change. It isn't just the pregnant partner who is undergoing an identity change; both of you are becoming new people and processing it in your own ways. Maybe it's okay and even good to connect over your shared anticipation as you get closer to the event that will transform you—as individuals and as a unit. And once parenthood is upon you, there will be less time for each other than there was before. Newborns don't do a whole lot, but somehow they eat up a ton of attention and affection, and it might be a while before you can access the ways you used to connect with your partner: regular date nights; weekend getaways; uninterrupted conversations.

This doesn't mean you're getting it wrong. It doesn't mean your marriage is doomed or on the brink of failure. We're given this well-intentioned advice to always put our marriages first, but I wonder whether that's simply impossible to do with a new baby in the house, especially if one partner is primarily responsible for the feeding or caregiving. I think what's under the advice is the idea that we shouldn't lose sight of each other amid the upheaval. When it feels like we're lost at sea in the middle of a storm, we may not be able to hold hands all the way through, but we can work in tandem to survive it. We can lock eyes in the middle of the maelstrom and swim toward each other once the winds calm.

Regardless of what's ahead for our partnerships, we can always turn to each other on the couch or at the restaurant or in the car, letting our exhausted selves meet for a moment, saying without words, "I'm here with you now. And I'll find you again."

22

Aches and Pains

My body had changed again, seemingly overnight. Suddenly, I couldn't lie on one side longer than an hour or two without needing to roll over and relieve the pain in my hip, and I couldn't roll over without grunting my way through a three-point turn. My shoulders, hips, and back ached when I got out of bed, and the only source of relief was a hot shower. My workout routine, which used to be energizing, left me sore in all the wrong ways. Instead of the welcome, empowering sensation of muscle fatigue, I felt flashes of lightning in my pelvis, tenderness in my core, and increasing tightness in my sciatic nerve.

Even my once-relaxing evening routine suffered from the changes: once I finally settled into the perfect position on the couch, my legs would grow restless. The internal itchiness started in my feet and spread up my calves like a swarm of ants, driving me toward a new understanding of what people mean when they say they want to crawl out of their skin.

There's no escape, at least until our babies are born. We can't take off our pregnant bellies at the end of the day like we can a pair of uncomfortable jeans or an ill-fitting underwire bra. And often the thing that would usually provide our bodies with the healing and restoration they need—a good night of sleep—also becomes unavailable because of the discomfort.

All this new pain, all at once, left me feeling at odds with my body.

Over the previous few years, I had experienced unwelcome pain and injury. While training for a race, I ramped up my running mileage too quickly and overused my IT band. Another time, I missed a step outside my apartment and rolled my ankle. At work, I slipped on a wet floor and hit my head. In each incident, there was a clear cause, clear effect, and clear prescription: rest, rehabilitate, return to activity.

For my current condition, the cause and effect were clear enough: I was growing a human, so my joints were getting looser in preparation for labor and the weight of the baby was causing strain on my pelvis and spine. But I lacked a clear prescription—even with rest and rehabilitation, the baby would only continue to get bigger, exacerbating the aches and pains.

I switched to a gentler workout plan and tried some prenatal barre videos. The instructor frequently encouraged me to "listen to my body," a phrase I had heard before in fitness settings but usually ignored; it felt a little too woo-woo for me. I'd always been able to push past my perceived limits, and when my body felt tired or sore or sick, I would work harder to keep up my normal pace.

But in pregnancy, my body refused to be ignored. It started with the exhaustion and nausea in the first trimester and continued with the weight gain I needed but couldn't control. As the baby took up more space and changed my center of gravity, my body signaled for attention again. My daughter grew stronger, flexing her muscles within me and ramping up her movement, and my own movement necessarily had to slow down. I had to stop resisting and start listening.

Perhaps what I wanted most was for my body to feel like it was mine again, like it was recognizable in its form and function. But would it ever? My body was being stretched now, further than it had ever been stretched, and soon it would be broken open for my child and given up for her comfort and sustenance in the aftermath.

It's always hard for humans to accept our limitations. We stay up too late because we resent the fact that we need sleep; we constantly add to our to-do lists because we feel pressure to do it all; we push ourselves to be more, achieve more, acquire more, because *more* always seems *better*. And usually, our endeavors end in burnout, which is essentially the forced acknowledgment that we are merely humans, who have amazing but limited bodies.

During pregnancy specifically, our bodies change in ways we can't predict, ways that are often painful and unpleasant and bring constraints we haven't faced before. We may instinctually perceive these new limits as evidence that our bodies are working against us. But really, our bodies are working *on behalf of someone else*. They no longer exist only to serve us but to provide a nourishing, protective home for our children. Our bodies know how to do this intuitively, but it takes our minds some time to catch up.

The nine and a half months of pregnancy, and the intensive season of mothering that comes after it, can feel like one long wrestling match: with ourselves, with our fear, with our changing bodies, even with God. We wrestle with the loss of how things used to be and with the fear and anticipation of how life will look after. We wrestle with our emotions when we feel both grateful and overwhelmed, when we experience joy and grief in the same breath. We wrestle with this new version of ourselves, one that is not yet complete, one that will change again after our babies are born. And in the process, we sustain stretch marks and scars, wider hips and looser skin, aching backs and new perspectives.

We will never be the same; we will always be marked by motherhood. If our hearts and souls are forever altered by the process of becoming mothers, then of course our bodies will be changed forever too.

But that doesn't mean we have to suck it up and enjoy every minute of the process.

One day at work, about halfway through my third trimester, I was commiserating with my friend Nicole, who was also pregnant and a few weeks further along than I was. We were comparing our physical and emotional pain points and taking solace each time the other person gasped and said, "Me too!" After we'd shared a litany of complaints, Nicole's expression visibly changed from exasperated to enlightened.

"You know what," she said, her eyes shining with her new discovery, "we don't have to be heroes. There's no trophy at the end of this, besides the baby. Let's take Tylenol. Let's ask our husbands for back rubs. Let's admit now that we want the epidural."

I don't have to be a hero. This was a new and novel concept for me, and it became my mantra for the rest of pregnancy.

Yes, my body was changing rapidly, and it hurt, and it was hard. Yes, there was more pain to come during labor and recovery, and that felt daunting. But I didn't have to be a hero, and you don't have to be a hero either. We can let our pain be productive, reminding us of the way our bodies are making space for our children.

In its most basic form, pain is a signal from our bodies to pay attention because something is happening here. We can both soothe our pain and be mindful of it, learning to have compassion and respect for our bodies in the process. We can care for ourselves and also revel in what our pain is producing, knowing it is charting the course to meeting our children. We can listen and respond to our bodies, trusting they are working in our best interests and in the interests of our babies.[5]

And we can be really, really grateful that pregnancy doesn't last longer than forty-two weeks.

---

5 Not all pain is productive, of course. It can stem from other health issues, or it may be unexplainable, or it may be long-term—something you dealt with before pregnancy and something you expect to endure after. I deal with purposeless, chronic pain myself, and I still feel unqualified to make sense of it. What I'm talking about here are the "normal" aches and pains we experience in pregnancy.

23

Birth Plan

I watched as a nearly naked stranger bounced on a birthing ball, leaked amniotic fluid, grunted through contractions, and groaned in pain. I tried to reconcile my current experience with the one playing out on the screen in front of me. I was seated at a long table in a hospital class-room, which smelled of lemon cleaner and new carpet. My hair and makeup were done, and I was fully clothed and relatively comfortable, sipping my coffee as I watched these women experience the most intense pain of their lives.

If there was any doubt in my mind about whether to get the epidural, the videos from the labor and delivery class dissolved it. Could I give birth without pain-relieving drugs? Sure, probably. Women have been doing it for thousands of years, and I deeply respect the women who still choose this path. But did I *want* to give birth without pain-relieving drugs? No, thank you. Because of my friend Nicole, I was trying to absolve myself of being a hero in life, in pregnancy, and in childbirth. In my perfect birth scenario, I was numb from the waist down.

Since I assumed I would get an epidural, what did I really need to know about labor except how to recognize it was happening and when to go to the hospital? There was no need to commit to a childbirth method that required twelve weeks of classes. Besides, I had worked hard to create space for myself leading up to my daughter's arrival, and

I didn't want to give up multiple weekends to learn how to survive one day of labor. But it also seemed unwise to go into labor knowing nothing about the process. I figured taking a one-day childbirth class through my hospital would be a happy medium, and from there, the labor and delivery nurses would fill in the gaps as it was happening.

In this class, the instructor—a peppy nurse practitioner who was an experienced mother and grandmother—had given a brief overview of the phases of labor and what to expect in each, and then we watched videos of various women experiencing each phase. Though the instructor emphasized many times that most birth experiences don't follow the framework perfectly, she also reminded us that our bodies knew what to do.

I'd had a pretty textbook pregnancy so far, with only minor hiccups—the bleeding that had turned out to be normal and a low-lying placenta that had moved out of the way by thirty weeks. I had followed all the rules. I had learned to trust my body. I was carrying a healthy baby who was head down and ready to go. Certainly, I thought, my labor would continue the pattern: my body would do what it needed to do, at least loosely following the "rules" of labor, and I would go along for the ride—ideally, with the help of a catheter in my spine.

In the last few weeks of pregnancy, whenever I found myself falling back into anxious thought patterns, I would run through the phases of labor in my head and reflect on the instructor's words: *Your body knows exactly what to do.*

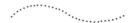

All my life, I have been an overplanner, overpacker, overpreparer, and overachiever.

For my wedding day, I created a timeline that was four pages long, single spaced. I broke the day down into fifteen-minute increments, with bullet points under each time slot detailing who would be where and what would be happening. The final page included a list of important names and phone numbers: three people who could field day-of questions, all my vendors, the entire wedding party, and our families. I emailed this document to the bridal party and vendors the week before the wedding, and I brought printed copies for everyone to the rehearsal.

When we took a vacation to Disney World, I planned every hour of every day in advance, set my alarm early on the day our FastPass+ booking window opened, and set up text alerts to notify me if a reservation opened up at a coveted restaurant. I sent the itinerary to everyone in our group and asked them to screenshot it and make it their phones' home screen. That way, we would never be without the master plan, even if my phone died.

I call this kind of behavior being prepared.

Some people might call it being controlling.

Maybe they're not wrong.

Deep in my bones, I believe if I plan for as much as I possibly can, I will maximize enjoyment and minimize disappointment. But it never fails that something goes wrong, or simply doesn't go according to my plan, and I struggle to be flexible and roll with the change. In an instant, my sky-high expectations come crashing down, and I experience the sting of disappointment. It clouds my memories of the otherwise special event, tingeing them with resentment and what-ifs. Attempting to stick to the plan at all costs doesn't minimize disappointment—it exacerbates it.

I had heard story after story from women who'd had very specific birth plans. One friend wanted an epidural, and then it was too late; another wanted a natural birth at the birthing center but had to be transferred to the hospital for a C-section; another wanted a scheduled C-section, and then her water broke two weeks early. I hadn't heard a single story in which birth went exactly according to plan. So I began to wonder: *If I can't control the process anyway, why set rigid expectations?*

I was weighed down by baggage from so many moments of disappointment over the years. People often say that when things don't go according to plan, it makes for a funny story or treasured memory later. Not for me. Even long after a disappointment, I don't laugh about it. I ruminate and regret and struggle to let it go.

It seems like there is a lot of cultural pressure to have the perfect birth, which feels odd to me because there's so little about childbirth that we can predict. To avoid defaulting to overplanning mode, I decided—maybe for the first time in my life—to stay out of my own way.

I gave myself permission to name a few things that would make birth feel ideal to me, acknowledge that those things might not happen, and get comfortable with the idea that there may be some grief along with the joy on that day. Besides, I truly believed my body intuitively knew how to give birth. My body didn't intuitively know how to plan a wedding or create a dream vacation, but surely, this baby was coming with or without a plan. Whichever way my daughter exited my body, however painful the process would be, I'd eventually have her tiny, wriggly body in my arms.

In my ideal birth, labor would come on spontaneously, I'd have an epidural, and the baby would be delivered vaginally. I was nervous about the possibility of a C-section because it's a major surgery and the recovery would be significantly longer and more painful.

I also hoped I wouldn't need to be induced, partially because I'd heard Pitocin can make the contractions even more excruciating than they are naturally. More than that, though, needing an induction would mean one of two things: one, something was wrong and I needed to deliver quickly, or two, I was overdue enough to require medical intervention to get the baby out of me. And to be honest, I still held on a bit to the fantasy of labor. I knew the movie depictions were inaccurate—a gush of water or a single contraction that comes out of nowhere, resulting in a rush to get to the hospital. But I did romanticize the idea of the contractions coming on slowly, timing them as they became more intense, and then looking at Dan and realizing *This is it!* as we grabbed our bags and drove to the hospital. And of course, I hoped Selah and I would be healthy through the whole experience.

I acknowledge that sometimes birth doesn't go according to even the bare-bones ideal of healthy baby, healthy mother. There may be complications we can't anticipate, NICU stays we can't foresee, tragedies we could never prepare for. But if I had let myself dwell on those possibilities, fear would have frozen me, and I'd had enough of fear in this pregnancy. I chose to believe the best because I couldn't allow myself to fear the worst anymore.

As I approached my due date, I tried to let go of even these expectations by focusing on what was true, however my daughter was born: I would hold my baby, eventually. I would heal, eventually. I would continue this extraordinary process of becoming a mother in the delivery room or in the operating room or in the car if we didn't make it to the hospital. Dan would be holding my hand as our baby was born and as we walked across the threshold of parenthood. And God would be with me through every pain, every push, and every moment when I thought I wouldn't be able to keep going—in the rest of my pregnancy and in the waves of labor and in the throes of new motherhood.

God is no stranger to the pains of bringing forth new life. Mary carried Jesus, the living God, in her womb, creating with God as she allowed the spirit to do its work in her, growing and sustaining and strengthening life. Her pregnancy was not at all what she had planned, and I imagine giving birth far from her home was not exactly how she had pictured this holy delivery playing out. But God chose this humble beginning for the incarnation. God chose to enter humanity the way we all do, via our mothers. God chose to be present not just in spirit but in *body* for the pain and brokenness and blood of birth.

Through our own experiences of pregnancy and birth—whatever they look like—we get to be cocreators and colaborers and cobirthers with God.

Maybe it's a gift that we don't have full control over how childbirth will happen. We can't decide we are ready for labor and flip a switch to get things going—which is a good thing, because many of us would likely never feel ready. (Done? Absolutely. But *ready* feels like a much higher bar than *done*.)

We aren't in charge of releasing hormones into our bloodstreams or opening our cervixes or making our babies descend. We are not bystanders to labor, but neither are we conductors. We are active participants, following the lead of our bodies, working in tandem with the God who groans life into being.

We don't have to engineer the miracle.

We get to be present for it.

24

An Early Advent

The final weeks of pregnancy can feel as long as the eight months that came before them. It's like waiting to take an exam you've prepared for, but you don't know the date you'll have to sit for it. And being overdue is a bit like expecting you'll sit for the test one day, only to have the date pushed back indefinitely.

It's a relief, in one way, because there is more time to prepare. It's a letdown, in another, because at some point you just want to get it over with.

The stakes are even higher as you wait for this life-changing event, one in which you will experience the most intense pain and joy of your life. It's a weird time warp that feels like you're somehow getting both closer to and further from the big event.

I had a week to go until my due date and had done all I could to prepare. The nursery was finished, the baby swing assembled, the car seat installed and double-checked by a safety technician. Labor class: check. Newborn care class: check. Hospital bag: check.

Just as I started to breathe a sigh of relief that I'd gotten it all done, that I finally felt ready for this baby to arrive, I felt a sore throat coming on.

I didn't think much of it—it's normal for me to get a sore throat when I'm exhausted, and being near the end of pregnancy was certainly exhausting. But in the following days my throat started to swell, and an intense pressure developed behind my eyes and cheeks, like my head was simultaneously filled with hot coals and also ready to float away. So I scheduled an appointment with a nurse practitioner at my doctor's office.

After a quick exam, she said everything looked normal but she would swab my throat just in case. Five minutes later, she checked the test strip and said, "Wow! Looks like you have strep after all!"

"I do? I've never had strep before in my life." I sat in disbelief on the exam table.

"Really? Not even as a kid?"

"Never," I said. "Bronchitis at least once or twice a year. But never strep."

"And you're how many weeks pregnant?" she asked, glancing once again at my beach-ball-sized belly.

"Thirty-nine."

"Well, that's some bad luck."

In an instant, I was no longer waiting eagerly for my daughter to make her appearance. I was waiting in dread: waiting for the antibiotics to kick in, waiting to feel better, waiting to see whether Dan would catch it. (He did.) My OB said if I didn't recover by the time Selah arrived, I would have to wear a surgical mask after she was born in order to protect her. The prospect of having a barrier between us gutted me, eager as I was to kiss her tiny cheeks and breathe in the delicious scent of her fresh newborn head—my reward for having carried her for nine months.

Instead of wishing I would go into labor soon, I hoped I would stay pregnant long enough to no longer be contagious, to recover my energy, and to be fully ready to embrace both the childbirth process and the round-the-clock work that would come after. As I waited, every minute felt like an hour; every hour, a day. I was stuck in the already and the not yet—empty time, as poet John O'Donohue calls it:

> *You have been forced to enter empty time.*
> *The desire that drove you has relinquished.*
> *There is nothing else to do now but rest*
> *And patiently learn to receive the self*
> *You have forsaken in the race of days. . . .*
> *Be excessively gentle with yourself.*[6]

I had been through the race of days, the flurry of activity leading up to the birth of a baby, and now all that was left to do was rest and be excessively gentle with myself. I tried to heed the advice of seasoned mothers to enjoy this time, to sleep and relax all I could, because it would be a long time before my days were totally mine again. I lay on the couch and binged *Jane the Virgin*. I called in sick to work when I couldn't focus on the computer screen. I made hot tea with honey and lemon and went to bed early.

It was an introvert's dream for the first few days. By day four, I was climbing the walls and wishing I felt well enough to get out of the house. By day six, my due date, I was feeling more like myself and ready to finally get this baby out.

Sick or not, I have a feeling those final few weeks would have brought up exactly the same feelings: wanting to savor the moments that were left of pregnancy while simultaneously wishing I could meet my baby already; trying to enjoy the baby's kicks while also wishing I could count her toes on the outside; trying to psych myself up for labor and believe it would begin at exactly the right time while also scouring the internet for tricks to get it started sooner.

---

6 John O'Donohue, "For One Who Is Exhausted," *To Bless the Space Between Us* (New York: Doubleday, 2008), 125-26.

Ten days after the positive strep test, I went to my OB for a cervical check and nonstress test, since I was past my due date. I'd been contracting on and off for a few days and thought for sure I'd made some early progress and labor might begin at any moment. I welcomed it: I felt fully recovered from the strep, and the size and weight of my belly were making me increasingly miserable. I had tracked my contractions at night a few times, thinking the real thing might be upon me. But every time, I fell asleep and woke up disappointed the next morning. The exam I had studied for had been delayed. I wasn't in labor.

Dr. Page checked my cervix and then told me gently that it was completely closed and very firm. My eyes filled with tears, and the doctor, sensing my frustration and disappointment, looked me in the eye and reminded me that a cervical check simply tells us the state of the cervix at this moment in time. It's not a great predictor of when labor will start.

"I've seen women who were dilated for the last four weeks of their pregnancies, and I've seen women who were closed up at their morning appointment and went on to deliver their babies that night," she assured me.

I cried the rest of my disappointed tears in the car. Even though I was closer than ever to meeting my daughter, after how long the past few weeks had felt, it seemed like I would never get there. Without much left to do, the days started to move about as quickly as a post-office line. I was on edge all the time, wondering whether my contractions were "real" yet, whether my water might break from the force of Selah's relentless kicking.

Each day that brought me closer to childbirth also brought me closer to the start of Advent, which would begin thirteen days after my due date. Advent is the church season leading up to Christmas, a time marked by waiting and preparing for God to arrive, incarnate in the form of a human baby.

Waiting for our babies to arrive feels a lot like a personal Advent: we know our lives are about to be divided forever into "before" and "after," but we don't know when the before will end or what the after will look like. We can't quite imagine how the transition will go, except we know it will be saturated with agony and expectation at a level we have not experienced before. This is what I find most mystifying about Advent: the period of waiting ultimately ends in great joy, but we can't get to that great joy without intense, active, unbearable pain.

In Advent we sense the mingling of anticipation and anxiety, excitement and disappointment, joy and pain, hope and fear. We ask ourselves, *Does God remember me? Does God understand me? Will God show up?* And as I waited for Selah to arrive, I asked myself those very same questions—and I wonder whether Mary did the same before Jesus was born.

I imagine her surprise pregnancy was the talk of her village, with people whispering about the scandal of it and doubting the story of this young girl. "Did you hear what she said?" they might have whispered behind their hands. "She claims she had a revelation from an angel!"

Did Mary feel lonelier than ever, wondering whether she'd heard right, whether she could trust her memory of that moment, whether this would all be worth it? *Does God remember me?*

I wonder whether she endured ridicule and scorn, whether her fellow villagers saw her coming and crossed to the other side of the road, whether her cheeks burned with shame and confusion. *Does God understand me?*

Mary then found herself a long way from home when it came time to deliver. Whether her waters released at once or her contractions became too intense to ignore, I don't know. But she knew it was time to labor, to push, to give birth to the one the world was expecting. *Will God show up?*

At the end of Advent, God answers our questions with a person: a baby wrapped in scraps of cloth and placed in a trough.

God shows up as Jesus, complete with a body—the vulnerable, dependent body of a newborn baby who can't even hold up his own head.

God becomes a human, choosing to enter the world the way every human does—first developed in the womb of his mother and birthed out of her at exactly the right time.

God remembers us in our time of transition, God remembers us right now, because God is present with us always. God is present in our breath, in the design of our bodies, in the season of waiting and the season of fulfillment.

The fulfillment of Advent is described in Galatians 4:4–5 (esv) this way: "When the fullness of time had come, God sent forth his son, born of a woman." The phrase "the fullness of time" makes me think of a fit-to-burst pregnant belly and a mom who is aching for sweet relief and longing to begin the next season of life. So often I want to skip ahead in my own waiting—to end the wait at the halfness of time, or the three-quarterness of time—because that last bit of waiting is the most painful of all. We've done all we can do. We've been stretched as far as we can stretch. We've waited as long as we have the patience for. And then we're called to wait some more.

Advent is that sacred space: the anticipation building in the space between pains, as we catch our breath and ready our bodies and souls for what's next. It is holy and hushed, active and alive, painful and promising. It takes work to wait well when it feels like time is standing still. But no matter how slowly time seems to be moving on the surface, its current is propelling us toward the main event—to the breaking and opening, the healing and resulting wholeness. Not by our own clocks or calendars but in the fullness of time.

We don't get to choose when our waiting will end, when our time of transition will arrive, when the work that has been started in us will finally be complete. In this final stretch, we may feel drawn to activity or rest, movement or stillness. We may wish to surround ourselves with friends or draw further inward.

However we choose to get through these final weeks, the ending to our waiting is remarkably similar. We will arrive at a moment when the past nine months reach a crescendo and our bodies break open to release life: the answer to our questions, the evidence dispelling our doubts, the reward for our waiting. In the fullness of time, the formation of our motherhood will crystallize, just for a moment, as we step into our much-anticipated *after*.

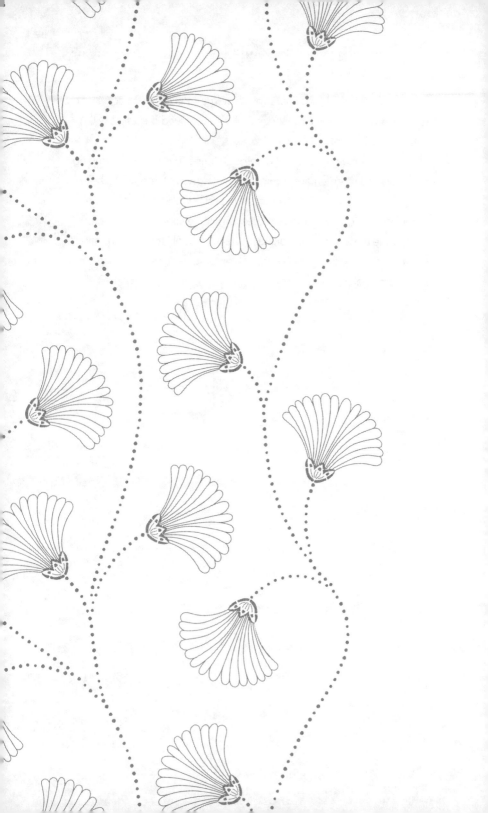

25

Birth

My doctor scheduled an induction for Black Friday, eleven days after my due date. I was to arrive at the hospital on Thanksgiving night for monitoring and administration of Cervidil (basically a tiny tampon that contains a drug to help soften and open the cervix), and then I would start Pitocin in the morning.

From the moment I learned that my due date was in mid-November, I had imagined what Thanksgiving would look like that year: Dan and I would spend the morning decorating for Christmas, stringing lights on the tree and listening to the crackle of a fire while our newborn snoozed in the baby swing. Later, our parents and siblings would arrive at our house bearing foil-covered casserole dishes, and we'd pass the baby around while eating forkfuls of turkey, mashed potatoes, and sausage stuffing.

On Thanksgiving, our family did arrive with all the fixings for a traditional holiday meal—more than enough to pack our fridge with leftovers—but that precious baby was still in my womb, with one more day to go of being carried by me alone.

We didn't have a dining table yet, so we all sat in mismatched chairs crowded around a long folding table, which my mother-in-law, Sharon, had draped in a plastic tablecloth bordered with cornucopias. Anticipation coursed through my body, making my stomach turn. I would be on a liquids-only diet in a few hours, though, so I ate as much as I could bear.

Sharon and my mom spoke excitedly about the baby, making predictions about who she would look like; Dan and his dad exploded with laughter over some joke I'd missed. Even as the noise rose steadily around me, I curled deeper and deeper into myself, feeling alone but not lonely, as if I were adrift on a raft in the middle of a placid lake.

Earlier that week, I had walked out of my doctor's office holding a small appointment-reminder card for the date of my induction— as if I could forget. Fear and resignation snaked their way into my chest as my hard-won trust in my body began to falter. My body hadn't, and probably wouldn't, go into labor on its own. I wouldn't have that revelatory moment when the contractions became too strong and too close together to stay home a moment longer. Though I had attempted to hold my expectations for labor loosely, this was one I'd clung to more tightly than I'd realized.

I tried to make peace with the idea of an induction: I let myself grieve that labor wouldn't look the way I'd always imagined, and I felt one finger uncurl from around my expectations. I asked friends to share their positive induction stories, and I felt another finger uncurl. I asked my doctor whether Pitocin contractions are really as bad as every-one says, and she said all contractions are that bad, it's just part of the deal, and another finger released. I considered how nice and normal it seemed to have a clear deadline, a date when I knew the baby would be here, and another finger loosened its grip. By the time Thanksgiving rolled around, I was willing to do almost anything to be free of my preg-nant body, to have my baby in my arms instead of pressing on my pelvis, my spine, and my hips. And with that, my hands were open again.

After dinner, our parents sent me to the couch to enjoy my last little bit of rest, and I listened to the hum of water filling the sink, the clink of silverware being dropped into a glass to soak, the click of containers being sealed and placed in the fridge. The air in the house was like a champagne bottle about to be uncorked; my loved ones were ready to bubble over with anticipation and excitement. My daughter kicked and sent a ripple of movement across the top of my belly, and I closed my eyes, willing her to come quickly. Neither of us had any concept of life on the other side, but we were together here, and we'd be together there too.

A few hours later, only my mom remained with us. Earlier, amid the activity, I had felt separate from it all—peaceful, or close to it—but now in the quiet of this moment, I pulsed with restless energy. I double- and triple-checked my hospital bag, until Dan gently took it out of my hands and loaded it into the car. I puttered around, moving piles of paper and baby gifts to new locations, not actually tidying anything but feeling desperate for something to do. My mom snapped a picture before we left, and when I look at it now, I see two genuine smiles betrayed by almost manic eyes. All we knew was that we didn't know what we were in for.

There was hardly any traffic on the road during our twelve-minute drive to the hospital. The sun had already set, our path lit by the glow of streetlamps and headlights, and I had the overwhelming sensation that we were diving deep into the belly of a beast and that everything along this familiar road would look different when we emerged.

"You're two centimeters dilated!"

I burst into tears, releasing the stress and pain and anxiety and excitement that had built in me over the last nine hours. My head sank further into the pillow as Dan stroked my hair.

"This is good news!" Dr. Page exclaimed. "Some women don't make progress on the Cervidil at all. Even half a centimeter counts. It shows that your body is ready for labor."

We had arrived at the hospital at eight o'clock the night before and checked in at the nurse's station, our suitcases in hand. An attendant showed us to our room as if we were at some sort of bizarre hotel.

A cervical check revealed I was one and a half centimeters dilated and 50 percent effaced, so the plan was to start with Cervidil. The nurse, Katie, advised me not to get my hopes up, because sometimes it works and sometimes it doesn't, and I shouldn't expect to go into labor until we started Pitocin. My doctor would be in at nine o'clock the next morning to check my progress, administer the Pit, and break my water. Katie held out an Ambien in one hand and a tiny plastic cup of water in the other and encouraged me to get some rest.

Even with the sleeping pill, I tossed and turned on the thin hospital mattress and dozed for only a few minutes at a time, until I felt a tightening in my belly . . . and then another one, and another. The episodes weren't terribly painful, and I remembered Katie saying I probably wouldn't go into labor that night. I tried to sleep it off like I had every other evening of the past few weeks, but these surges wouldn't be ignored.

I heard a knock on the door shortly after midnight, and Katie popped her head in. "Are you feeling those contractions?" She had been watching the monitor at the nurse's station and was surprised at how frequently they were coming.

"I am," I told her, a note of confusion in my voice. "They're not super painful, but they're keeping me up. Are they real? I thought labor wouldn't start until tomorrow."

"Yes, they're real. This baby might be coming sooner than we expected—your body just needed a little nudge."

Katie helped me get set up on a birthing ball, and I bounced by the side of the bed, watching episode after episode of *The Office* on my laptop while Dan slept. It would be better if we weren't both sleep deprived going into the next day, but as the pain intensified, so did my envy that he was sleeping so peacefully while I labored. I stood and swayed, got back on the ball, lay on my side, and all the while the contractions became stronger and stronger.

At first they had felt like mild period cramps, starting low in my abdomen and twisting a bit before releasing. But after a few hours they gained strength, gripping my belly and my back like an iron fist and squeezing the air out of my lungs. I had little break between each one, which confused and alarmed me.

I woke Dan when I could no longer handle the pain on my own. His presence coupled with the morning light trickling in through the window revived me. *I can totally do this*, I thought as the clock ticked closer to nine o'clock. *And since my contractions are already close together and have been for hours, I must be near the end.* In labor class I had learned that transitional contractions are less than two minutes apart, so logically, I had to be close to or in transition. The doctor would check me, and I would be at seven or eight centimeters. It might even be too late for the epidural.

I greeted Dr. Page cheerily a couple of hours later, eager to find out how much progress I'd made. She was pleased that I'd been laboring all night and said we might not even need to use the Pitocin. She snapped a sterile glove onto her hand and felt around for my cervix. Her fingers swept back and forth a few times, and I felt the prize within my reach. My baby was right there, just inches away from her hand, ready to arrive. She would be in my arms in an hour or two, at the most.

That's when Dr. Page made her delighted declaration that I had gone from one and a half to two centimeters in the last nine hours of work and darkness and pain.

I lost it. My weary body started to tremble as I cried, my tears falling hot and fast. With my voice shaking and my breath shuddering in my chest, I explained that the contractions had been close together all night, I was exhausted and had made a marginal amount of progress, and if I kept going at this rate, I'd never have the strength to get the baby out.

"Of course you're exhausted." Dr. Page placed a hand on my leg. "You know you can get the epidural anytime, right?"

"I can?" I asked. "I thought I had to wait until five or six centimeters, so labor doesn't stall."

"That's always a risk, especially when labor comes on naturally. But we'll start your Pitocin drip now, and if the epidural slows things down, we'll increase your dosage. You can relax, take a nap, and rebuild your strength for pushing later."

I took a minute to consider what she was saying. Was I quitting by getting the epidural so early? Was I a strong, capable, empowered woman if I got pain medication long before the halfway point? Was I failing at childbirth?

Then I heard Nicole's gentle and familiar voice, which quieted my other thoughts: *You don't have to be a hero.*

"Should I call the anesthesiologist?" Dr. Page pulled me back into the moment.

I nodded my consent.

"Alright then." She asked Anna, the new nurse on duty, to make the call and then turned back to me. "Let's go ahead and break your water. It'll make your contractions more intense and more productive."

A few seconds later, I felt a swift tug and then a gush of warm liquid, which soaked the bedding and pooled under me as I tried to wiggle away. Anna helped me up so she could change the sheets, the water trickling down my legs and creating a puddle around my feet. I felt the urge to apologize for getting the floor wet, and then I realized my fluids were far from the first this floor had seen. My urge to apologize was replaced by an urge to put on shoes.

A searing, hot wave of pain crested over my abdomen, folding my body in half. My arms stretched toward the bed for support and a sound I'd never made before—a deep, primal moan—rolled out of my throat. As the wave receded, I lumbered into the bed to start my pre-epidural IV fluids, and less than two minutes later another wave crashed over me, and then another and another, leaving me pummeled and disoriented and shaken to my core.

So that's what real contractions feel like. I glanced at the clock: 9:15 a.m.

With every contraction I felt the pressure building in my body, tightening my abdomen, pulling me down into darkness. I closed my eyes and tried to imagine the place where I felt most alive, most at peace: the ocean. I pictured myself floating, paddling forward as I felt a wave rising behind me, riding it out as it propelled me to shore, feeling the welcome relief of the sand under my feet when it deposited me on land.

In between contractions, I imagined floating on my back, my body weightless in the water, the sun warming my skin. I held Dan's hand but felt more alone than ever, and I desperately wished I could drag him into the water with me.

Visualization provided a necessary distraction as I waited for the anesthesiologist, but it did nothing to quell the intensity of the waves, nothing to pacify the gut-wrenching pain that was blooming and then exploding out of me. I steeled myself against every contraction, tried to drum up every bit of strength and power and gumption left in my body, and willed myself to produce more energy and more fight. I imagined my hormones working like tiny bees, frantically trying to keep up with the demand for more.

I gritted my teeth, squeezed Dan's hand, crunched myself forward, and growled through the pain. My breath was ragged and disjointed, a primitive prayer.

Just after ten o'clock, help arrived in the form of a needle in my spine, administered by a woman I remember only in glimpses: the short, sandy hair that reminded me of Ellen DeGeneres, the black Nikes that squeaked as she walked around gathering her materials, the hearty laugh and gentle pat she gave me when my whole body wilted with relief and I told her deliriously that she was the restorer of life.

Dan and I had switched roles; he watched *The Office* while I dozed, my body finally at rest, the epidural seeming to drain the tension out of me more than pump medication into me. Dr. Page woke me around noon and asked whether I wanted a cervical check now or in a few hours. I didn't expect much out of it, but I wanted to know if I'd made any progress, even a little bit, to keep me going, to keep me believing I was moving forward now that I couldn't feel anything for myself.

When she announced I was at eight centimeters, I thought I was hallucinating, that the trip from the depth of pain to the height of relief had left me in shock, like stepping into a sauna after having been stuck in a polar vortex. I was dizzy, incoherent, imagining things.

"You're at eight centimeters," she repeated. "All you needed to do was relax. I could tell when I came in this morning that you'd been fighting. You were resisting. It's a normal thing to do in the face of this kind of pain, but it's not helpful. I knew if we got you the pain meds, your body would carry you the rest of the way."

I tried to follow along as she continued: "At this rate, you should be at ten centimeters within the hour, but I'm not going to have you push yet. Baby is pretty high, and your legs are so numb that pushing will be unproductive. It'll tire you out. You get some more sleep, wait for baby to descend, and let some of the medication wear off. When you start to feel your legs again, or if you feel the urge to push, let your nurse know, and she'll page me. Otherwise I'll check you again in a few hours."

I lay back in disbelief, still trying to process what Dr. Page had said.
I resisted.
My body carried me.
I'm almost there.
She's almost here.

I tried again to nap and was mostly unsuccessful, startling awake every time my eyelids got heavy. This time, it wasn't the pain keeping me up; it was the excitement that my body was working, that this would all be over soon, that my daughter was so close to being in my arms.

By four o'clock in the afternoon, I still couldn't feel my lower body, but I was growing impatient and didn't want to wait anymore. Anna had me try a few practice pushes, coaching me through each attempt. She and Dan each held a leg, and Dan stood in front of me holding a towel in his free hand. Every time a contraction rumbled within me, I was to take a deep breath, use the towel to pull myself up, and push with all my strength for a count of ten.

Anna pressed her fingers to the bottom of my vaginal opening and said, "Try to push right here, right where my fingers are." I heaved myself up and pushed again, but it was difficult to push properly when I couldn't feel anything below my chest. But I wasn't willing to stop now. I was on the edge of the biggest moment of my life, and I needed to *do* something, to usher this labor to its finale, to see my daughter's face and count her toes.

The three of us fell into a rhythm: legs back, breathe in, pull up, push hard, rest; legs back, breathe in, pull up, push hard, rest. Over and over I pushed, and when I glanced at the clock, I realized I'd been at it for close to an hour, without much change in the baby's position.

"You just need to get her head over your pubic bone," Anna said. "After that, she'll come out easily. I'll be able to see her head, and then I'll call in the delivery team."

That became my sign: once Anna called in the delivery team and the doctors, the end would be within reach. I would make it.

The epidural finally started to wear off, and I could feel impressions of pain, sensations of twisting and tightening. I welcomed it, knowing it was a signal I could listen to, a guide that would lead me to the finish line. But with the increase in pain came an increase in exhaustion. I begged

Anna to let me rest for a few contractions, and the mental switch from work to rest released a flood of emotion.

I couldn't imagine summoning the strength to finish. It had been hours since I'd had even a sip of water, and my throat felt raw every time I took a breath. The ice chips provided momentary relief but no sustenance. Loneliness consumed me.

"I can't do this," I whispered to Dan. I felt my whole self sag—my body, my mind, my spirit. I wanted to sink into the earth and allow the pain to bury me. A tender lump lodged itself in my throat, and fresh tears burned in my eyes. "I wish I could die instead."

My own words resonated somewhere deep inside myself, as if I had heard them before, or spoken them before. And then I remembered: in every birth story I'd ever heard, the mother reached a point where death seemed more attractive than continuing to live through labor. I felt an electric connection to the women who had been here before. It was a rite of passage, grim and hopeful at once—my turn to reach the end of myself, an act of sacrifice to face down death for the sake of my child.

In a last-ditch effort to renew my energy, I pictured these women surrounding me—my friends, my family, women from all over the world and from all eras of history, a sisterhood of mothers. I imagined their faces, remembered they had all reached the point of preferring death to life when they were drowning in pain, and reminded myself that they had found a way to rise back to the surface. Because they had done it, I could do it too.

Another contraction began to roll through me, gaining speed and intensity. I pushed again, gathering energy from the women I felt cheering me on, drawing on the shadows of strength left in my body.

"That's it! You're doing it! That's exactly right!" Anna shouted. The wave subsided and she looked me in the eye: "A few more pushes like that one and she'll be out!"

Her words filled me with a fresh burst of energy, and on the next contraction I pulled myself up higher, crunched over harder, pushed all the power down and out.

"I can see her head now! A full head of hair, the same color as yours, Mom!"

I fell back onto the pillow and started weeping.

Another rumble, another rise, another push.

"She's almost there! Let's get the delivery team in here!"

I made it.

The tears fell faster, my gentle cries of relief turning to sobs of bewilderment.

Here she comes, I thought. *The end of my before. The beginning of my after.*

Technicians bustled around the room and set up tools on the warming station. Dr. Page returned and scrubbed her hands, then slipped into a gauzy yellow delivery gown.

"This is it," she said. "Are you ready to meet your daughter?"

"Yes," I said, no louder than a breath. "Yes."

She pulled a surgical mask over her mouth and told me to push at half strength on the next contraction.

It had taken everything in me to push as hard as I could in the last few minutes, and now it took everything in me to hold back. I wanted to charge ahead and end the agony, but I let my body stretch and adjust and take its time.

"She's crowning now!" I heard Dr. Page's voice, muffled by her mask. "Two more pushes, Mom, nice and slow!"

My daughter's head came free on the first; on the second, her shoulders slipped out along with the rest of her body, and suddenly I was empty. All the pressure had drained out of me in one final gush of blood and water and baby.

The next thing I remember, my squirmy, slippery, seven-pound newborn was on my chest.

The edges of my vision narrowed, like a photo with heavy vignetting, and my whole body shook with relief and exhaustion and shock, tears mingling with sweat and slipping off my nose and my cheeks, sliding into the folds of my neck. A hand pressed down on my abdomen to help deliver the placenta, the doctor requested tools, assistants handed them over, but it was all happening to someone else. The only people in the room were my daughter and me.

This child had been inside me mere seconds ago, and now she was curled against my skin. Her magnetism seized me; though she was sticky with blood and vernix, I kissed her head, her ears, her fingers.

She lifted her head slightly, as much as her fragile neck muscles would allow, and locked her eyes on mine, searching me with a curiosity and an intensity I didn't know a newborn could exhibit. It was like she was daring me to take her on, asking whether I was ready for what she had in store for us.

I exhaled and pressed my lips to her skin again, whispered her name against her cheek: *Selah*.

26

After

I startled awake, panic exploding through my chest. For a fraction of a second, I had no idea where I was or why my limbs felt like they were filled with sand. My hand grabbed for the plastic rail of the hospital bed, and my heartbeat began to settle as I wiped away the beads of sweat that had started to form along my hairline. I checked the time on my phone and saw that I'd been asleep for less than two hours.

Morning light flooded in through the windows, creating pools of gold on the warm wood floors. I heard the faint scrape of metal as Dan pushed aside the curtain at the front of our hospital room, and then he entered, pushing a plastic bassinet that contained a tightly swaddled bundle. He explained that he'd brought Selah into the hallway to do some laps when she started to cry. The motion had worked to calm her, but every time he stopped moving, she would cry out again.

I pushed myself upright—no small task while sitting on a melted ice pack and a maxi pad the size of a pool raft—and then packed some pillows around me and reached my arms out for the baby. *My daughter.* I unclipped my nursing tank as she searched hungrily, primally, for food. Her mouth reminded me of a tiny barracuda's, and I gasped in pain as she latched onto my breast. I gently pulled her bottom lip out as the nurse had shown me.

I leaned my head back on my pillow as I thought about all that had happened in the past thirty-six hours. The contractions starting unexpectedly at midnight. The loneliness of laboring while the world slept. The utter exhaustion and defeat when I learned I'd progressed only half a centimeter in those nine long overnight hours. The breathtaking intensity of the first surge after my water broke. The dread I felt every time a subsequent wave rose from within. The contractions growing stronger and stronger until a needle in my spine melted the pain.

I had thought my body would intuitively know what to do in labor. And perhaps it did, but I didn't account for the fact that on some level, despite how much I'd learned and grown during pregnancy, I still thought I needed to objectify my body, master it, subdue it—that I was separate from it, or at least independent of it. Labor, through that lens, was happening *to* my body, and it was my job to fight against the pain.

But labor wasn't some outside force acting upon me; it was arising from *within* me. The pain was not pointless or punishing, something I needed to oppose; it was a creative, productive process I needed to give myself to. The only way to survive the pain was to find a way to work *with* my body to deliver my daughter.

Selah's suckling slowed as she drifted off to sleep again, and I whispered to Dan to come take her so I could use the restroom. I peeled back the blankets and gingerly moved one leg and then the other off the side of the bed, placed my hands on the mattress, and lifted myself up, trying not to drag my stitches. My knees threatened to buckle as I stood up, but then my muscles began firing, waking up as I shuffled to the bathroom. It was less than ten feet away but felt like a hundred yards.

I closed the door behind me and found myself looking in a mirror for the first time since Selah was born. My hair was matted and shiny with oil; my eyes were ringed with circles so dark it looked like I had rubbed mascara onto the papery skin; my belly was a deflated dodge-ball, the skin loose and squishy and lined with purple stretch marks I hadn't noticed before.

Everything hurt, and I had never looked quite as shell-shocked or tired as I did at that moment. But what I felt when I looked in the mirror was not disgust or horror or even pity. As I studied the belly that had housed my child for nine and a half months and felt my legs shaking from my effort to push her into the world, I felt pride rushing from my toes to my chest. My body was no longer my personal object, but my friend; no longer an *it*, but a *she*. And she had been my guide and my partner through the most harrowing experience of my life.

When the anesthesiologist had guided the needle into my back twenty-four hours earlier, I wondered whether I was giving up too soon. Maybe I should have fought longer, tried harder. My doctor's grace-filled words floated into my head: *All you needed to do was relax. I knew if we got you the pain meds, your body would carry you the rest of the way.*

As with so many other moments in my life and in this pregnancy, I'd had to get out of my own way, to learn from my body instead of trying to control her. And when I did, she took over exactly the way she was supposed to. She had known what to do all along, even in my panic that labor wasn't going according to plan, even when I didn't trust her to survive it at all, let alone have the stamina to get the baby out successfully. I had thought she was working against me, ripping me apart one contraction at a time. But once I stopped fighting—albeit with the help of a numbing agent—she opened up, making way for the baby she had grown, as if to say, *See? I've got this. Trust me.*

I had resisted and then succumbed, been a fighter and then a bystander. And when it came time to push, I knew what I had to do: join my body and become an active participant.

Legs back, breathe in, pull up, push hard, rest; legs back, breathe in, pull up, push hard, rest.

Over and over until I reached the end of my strength and abilities, when I became too tired to pull myself up and push even one more time, when I was on the brink of a breakdown and wishing for death, when I'd been pushing for an hour and the baby still wasn't descending.

Just when it all felt hopeless—the sun setting on a full day of labor, plunging the room into darkness—the sisterhood of mothers reminded me that *this is how it is done*. This is how it has always been done, bringing new lives into the world. Whether spontaneously or by induction, whether assisted with pain relievers or all natural, whether on a delivery table or an operating table, there is always work and pain, reaching the end of what we think we're capable of and then needing to dig deeper.

Another push, and a glimpse of hair. Another push, and her crowning head. Another push, another push, another push, and then I was torn open.

Blood and fluid spilled out of me, a baptism of sorts. I had reached the end of myself and desired death, and in a way, I'd had to let myself die in order to be delivered: from my expectations, from my need for control, from my desire for perfection, from my sense of shame. It all came surging out of me as my body and my life were torn down the middle. Before and after. Then and now. Death and life.

And then a final push, gentler than the others, delivered two new people into the room: a fresh baby, a brand-new mother.

I rinsed my most tender areas with warm water, applied pain-relieving cream, and stepped into a clean pair of mesh underwear lined with an ice pack. This would become my liturgy in my first weeks as a mother: tending to the places where I had been broken and stitched up, being gentle with myself through the pain, moving slowly as I learned to care for two people at once.

In some moments I was afraid of my ravaged body—I desperately wanted to feel normal again and couldn't imagine I ever would. Her wounds were too deep, the changes too profound. In other moments, I loved her—it felt right that an experience like childbirth would leave its mark, that she would need time to recover, that she wouldn't bounce back right away.

I washed and dried my hands and then stepped out of the bathroom. I heard visitors chatting outside the door, machines beeping their melody, a food cart being rolled down the hall, likely bearing sustenance for a fellow new mom. Dan was holding Selah by the window, the sunlight creating a golden glow around their profiles.

I got back into bed, and Dan placed Selah in my lap. I removed her swaddle blanket for some skin-to-skin time, my movements slow and deliberate as I tried not to disturb her too much. But as soon as the cold hospital air reached the bare skin of her legs, she started to wail, and I felt an instinctual desire to fix it. I settled her onto my chest, draped the blanket over us, whispered in her ear, *It's okay now. Mommy's here. You're safe.* Her knees curled into her chest as they had been in the womb, and her body released the tension that had built with her cries. She breathed in the scent of my skin, already familiar and comforting to her, and I leaned down to breathe in the scent of her head.

The fact of her existence had made me a mom, but it wasn't only the moment of her delivery that had minted me. It was the convergence of a thousand individual moments: the decision to try; the second pink line; speaking the news aloud to my loved ones; my tears over a mis-carriage scare; her jelly-bean body on the ultrasound; the sickness and exhaustion; the baby-shower celebrations and lonely late-night worry sessions; the nursery I prepared and the space I made; the fear and the growth; the pain and the change and the deliverance.

When I look back at photos taken of us in the hospital, I'm most drawn to my eyes. In one photo, I'm looking down at Selah, asleep in my arms, my gaze full of wonder and delight and affection. In another, I'm smiling with my whole face, radiating joy, my eyes tired but unmis-takably alive.

If the eyes are the window to the soul, then mine were wide open, revealing a version of me that had never existed before.

Mother. Mommy. Mom.

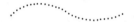

The next morning, Dr. Page checked on Selah and me one more time and then cleared us for discharge.

"Are you ready for the comfort of home?" she asked.

I had been a mother for less than two days, and I had only ever been a mother in the hospital. Here, where a 24/7 nursing staff helped me feed and diaper my new baby. Here, where three meals a day were prepared and cleaned up by other people. Here, where supplies—diapers and wipes and Tucks pads—were replenished as if by magic every time they got low. Soon I would have to figure it out from home, without on-call professionals to guide me.

I felt simultaneously weak and powerful, clueless and capable. I still wasn't sure how I would rise to the responsibility of motherhood, but I knew for certain I could. And I was far from alone: my husband, my friends, my God, my body, and my intuition would all be trust-worthy partners.

Later that afternoon, Dan pulled the car around to the front of the hospital, and an orderly wheeled Selah and me down to meet him. He pushed me through the sliding doors, and a gust of wind danced across my face and through my hair. I stood up and blinked into the late-November sunlight. Everything felt louder, brighter, more vibrant, as if someone had bumped up the saturation on the whole world.

No one else seemed to notice the change. Cars zipped by on the road beyond the hospital parking lot. The orderly pushed the empty wheelchair back inside. An elderly couple carrying balloons walked past me toward the entrance.

Don't you see it? I wanted to ask. *Doesn't it all look different to you?*

Dan clicked Selah's car seat into its base, and I eased my sore body into the front seat. We began the familiar drive to our familiar home, and I had the sense of coming back after a long time away.

Sometimes when I get home from a vacation, I walk into my house and it feels as if everything has shifted slightly. It's always a little bigger than I remember, a little brighter, a little more lived-in. My memory of the house is a shadow; the reality of it is alive.

I had that same feeling as we drove home, as we passed our regular grocery store, as we turned onto our tree-lined street.

Everything was different, yet everything was as I'd left it.

It wasn't the world that had come alive.

It was me.

Epilogue

The Force of Love

On May 2, 2019, I became a mother again when I delivered my son, Eamon, into the world.

His arrival was redemptive in a number of ways: he was my rainbow baby after a miscarriage, and my postpartum experience with him was everything Selah's wasn't. I recovered easily, worried less, enjoyed the present more. Instead of wishing time away, I found myself wishing I could suspend us in amber. He's cooing next to me as I write this, a happy and active four-month-old, and already I am nostalgic for the days when he would curl up on my chest and fall asleep.

I learned how to be a mom while carrying and caring for Selah: I learned how to feed her, how she liked to be held, how long she could handle being awake between naps, what purées she preferred and which ones she would spit out. I learned how to change diapers in just about any location—on the backseat of a car, on my lap during a flight—and how to carry seventeen bags plus an infant car seat. I learned how to function on little sleep and how to take care of myself.

In the period following her birth, I also discovered who I am as a mother: I am thoughtful and present and attentive. I become overstimulated by ten in the morning and desperately need a few minutes alone. I worry about my daughter every day. My biggest desire for her is that she feel secure in my love and safe in my presence.

Perhaps most important, during our first three years together, I learned how to come up for air while caught up in a love that devoured me, how to fight my way back to the surface and reclaim my sense of self.

And then I became a mother of two, and I've had to learn how to be a mom all over again. I remembered how to breastfeed, but I'm learning how to do dinner and bedtime solo with two kids when Dan works late. I remembered how to swaddle, but I'm learning what Eamon specifically needs to be ready for sleep. I remembered how to care for myself when I reach my limits, but I'm learning that my limits have changed and I have new warning signs when I'm approaching them.

I'm still in the all-consuming phase of new motherhood, in which my love for this child is somehow ferocious and primal and impossibly tender. This love has lodged itself into my heart, my gut, my brain; it follows me around all day, my thoughts shifting toward him constantly: *When was the last time he ate? Does he need a nap? Is he breathing? Does he want to be held?*

Above where Eamon is playing there is a window, and through it I can see a tree in the backyard that is bent over at nearly a 45-degree angle. Perhaps the tree grew this way from the start, but I like to think the wind kept blowing it in the same direction, and over time, the tree acquiesced.

Many days I feel like that tree: reoriented by the force of a love I cannot control.

Before my sister was born, I had a tearful conversation with my mom about what our lives would look like after the baby arrived. My brother was born when I was not quite three, and I had been too young to fully make sense of his birth. But this time I was eight—old enough to be aware that the family dynamics would change, and so would my mom's time and attention.

I was struggling to explain how I felt, so I grabbed a piece of paper and a red crayon, drew a small heart, and divided it in half. "Right now I have this half," I said, pointing to one side, "and Colin has this half. Since you're having a girl, my half is going to get cut in half again." I drew a line down my side of the heart. "Colin still gets half of your love, but I get half of half."

My mom pulled me in for a tight hug as I started to cry, and she assured me that this is not at all how a mother's love works. She flipped the paper over and drew a heart so massive it took up the entire page. Then she divided it into three roughly equal pieces.

"When you become a mom, or when you have a second or a third baby, your heart gets bigger. You don't have the same amount of love to divide into smaller and smaller pieces. Each piece gets bigger, because your whole heart gets bigger. I'm going to share my love with this new baby, but my love for you is going to get bigger too."

What I couldn't understand yet is a mother's love is not finite; it is boundless. Likewise, our identity as a mother is not one additional piece of who we are; it transforms everything else.

I used to think motherhood would be like adding an element to my life and my identity. I was already a daughter, a sister, an editor, a writer, a wife, and a friend. I would simply tack "mom" on to the list. The mom slice of my identity might be bigger than the other pieces, and it might grow or shrink over time, depending on the needs of my kids and the seasons of their lives. But everything would be neat and tidy, with clear boundaries. I would go to work, or go on a date with Dan, or get up early in the morning to write, and in those moments, I would take a break from being Mom. But it turns out my identity as a mother can't be so easily cordoned off.

Nothing about motherhood has been neat or tidy or predictable. For me, motherhood isn't a piece of the pie; it is the whole pie dish. Put another way, it's a lot like moving into a new house.

In preparation for the move, or the identity shift, I purged what I didn't want to take with me: fear and perfectionism, disconnection from my people and my body, the need to control everything. (Some of that stuff came with me anyway, sneaking into boxes I thought I had sealed.) I brought along my most treasured items but had to find new places for them to belong, and it took trial and error and time. Some pieces of myself are boxed up and gathering cobwebs in the basement, waiting to be opened and used once again, or released once and for all.

But motherhood, unlike these other parts of myself, isn't something I can pack and unpack when it suits me. Motherhood is the whole house, the frame that holds all the pieces of myself.

(By the way, motherhood isn't the only thing that can function as a house in our lives—for some, it might be a relationship or a career or a faith or an idea, or a combination of these, that provides a frame.)

I am more than motherhood, of course. I can leave the house, but the house always belongs to me, and it is the place I always return to. Sometimes I find a deep sense of satisfaction in this home, and other times I chafe against its boundaries.

It takes time to get used to a new house: We stumble around in the dark while trying to find the bathroom. We might arrange and rearrange furniture, trying to find the balance of beauty and efficiency. It takes a while to remember where the light switches are, which drawer holds the kitchen towels, which hinges creak and need oil.

But over time, through living in this space one day at a time, it begins to feel like home. I remember which stuffed animal my daughter can't sleep without, that my son needs help finding his thumb when he's falling asleep, that when my daughter is having a meltdown it usually means she is craving connection. Tasks that seemed impossibly difficult in the early months—feeding or calming or getting out the door— become second nature, things I could do in the dark. It has been painful and disorienting, but I've grown accustomed to this new house.

Sometimes you'll think about the old house, or your old self, and feel an undercurrent of grief. It was familiar and comfortable; you knew its intricacies and corners, how it all worked and where everything was. You may wonder whether you'll ever finish unpacking all the boxes, ever stop discovering how to live in this new place, ever feel comfortable and at home. Frustration will flare when you stub your toe on a corner you aren't used to, when you bump up against an obstacle you don't know how to move through. You might wish to return to what was, mourning all that was lost in the change: The time you used to have for yourself, for your partner, for your friends. The single-mindedness you could bring to a task. The functionality of your body. The feeling of being answerable primarily to yourself.

Other days, you'll marvel at how this new house can hold all this life, all this goodness, all this love and joy and wonder.

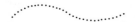

Unlike a new house, however, motherhood is not something we ever fully arrive at. There is no such thing as capital-M Motherhood. When we first saw those two pink lines, it kick-started a process that will only ever continue.

During pregnancy, it often feels like this process is happening outside of our control, but we are not passive recipients of the change. The very act of giving our consent, of allowing our children to make their first home in our bodies, sets us up to be partners in the journey to and through motherhood.

In Scripture, we see God using pregnancy to get the attention of God's people, to invite them to participate in something new, to help them arrive at a fresh understanding of who God is and what God is doing in the world.

Eve becomes pregnant and gives birth, the first woman to do so, and she declares, "With the Lord's help, I have *produced* a man," reminding us of her active role in the creative process (Genesis 4:1 NLT, emphasis added).

Sarah becomes pregnant when she's well past childbearing age and after decades of infertility. Nearly two thousand years later, Elizabeth, a relative of Mary's, becomes pregnant, also when she's very old and after a long period of infertility. And then we come to Mary, pregnant at the same time as Elizabeth. Mary is on the other end of the spectrum: she is incredibly young, a teenager at the very beginning of her childbearing years.

In each of these stories, God uses a process that is common—all humans grow inside of and are born from their mothers—to evoke a deep sense of surprise. God captures the attention of the mother and also points to something God is doing in the world at large. Sarah's pregnancy is the fulfillment a promise God made to her and her husband, Abraham, that they would produce a whole nation of people. Elizabeth's son will proclaim that God is coming to us. Mary's son *is* God incarnate, the truest picture of God the world has ever seen.

Over and over, God empowers women's bodies to announce God's goodness and nearness.

Through these brave women, we see that pregnancy is at once deeply personal and universally significant. Because of it, we are changed individually and profoundly. Through it, we participate in an ancient act that ties us to billions of women across time. In it, we create with God, bringing forth the next generation, and the next, and the next.

In Mary's story, the angel tells her, "Behold, you will conceive in your womb and bear a son, and you shall call his name Jesus" (Luke 1:31 ESV). Some versions translate *behold* as "listen," connoting a sense of "Listen up! Don't miss this!" The word for *conceive* means "to assist, to take part."

This, then, is the invitation: Allow God to capture your attention. Listen to what your body is saying. Don't miss the miracle happening in you and through you. Make space for change. Participate in this act of creation.

Embody creation.

As you become this new person, you may feel like your old self is crumbling before your eyes, like the pieces are being absorbed by the needs of another human. As your body and priorities and outlook change, you may lose sight of the *you* that you used to be.

Be assured that God is present with you in every one of these changes, inviting you to be part of the process, enabling you to reflect God's image as a sustainer. God's mother-love is shaping you, not into a generic mother but into *your* child's mother, the mother only you can be.

I hope you will make time and space to dwell in the change— in the moments that are exciting and full of hope, and also in the moments that are painful and jarring. I hope you will give yourself the tenderness you deserve. I hope you will thank your body, your mind, your spirit, and your heart for seeing you through the tumult. I hope you will surrender wholeheartedly to the transformation, even when you're not sure how everything is going to look on the other side. I hope you will awaken to yourself as you become someone new.

Mary responded to the angel with these now-famous words: "May it happen to me" (Luke 1:38 BSB).

May it happen to us, too, with our eyes and bodies and hearts wide open.

May we work with God to create new life and our new selves.

May we never stop marveling at the transformation.

May we never stop bending to the force of love.

May we never stop expecting wonder.

Acknowledgments

They say it takes a village to raise a child, and it also takes a village to birth a book. This one had many doctors, doulas, and caregivers, literal and metaphorical. I am deeply grateful to every person who helped give this dream life.

To my editor, Lisa Kloskin: Thank you, thank you, thank you for your enthusiasm for this book and for pushing me to make it the best it could be. I'm so grateful for every phone call, email, and thoughtful comment. Your edits have clarified my thinking, sharpened my writing, and strengthened my faith.

To the whole team at Broadleaf, especially Claire Vanden Branden, Mallory Hayes, Emily Benz, Madeleine Vasaly, and Lindsey Owens: Thank you for all the love and creativity you have poured into this book. I'm so thankful for your commitment to inclusivity, excellence, and thoughtful dialogue.

To my agent, Rachelle Gardner: Thank you for believing in me as a writer, being a trustworthy guide and advocate in this process, and finding a perfect home for this book.

To my second-grade teacher, Mrs. Arbo: Your affirmation of my first "memoir" ignited the writerly fire in my heart, and it's still burning bright. I'll always be thankful to you.

To so many friends and writing companions, far too many to name here, who encouraged me to go for it at every step along the way. Special thanks to the Exhale community and Redbud Writers Guild, to Stephanie Rische and Kara Leonino for showing me the way, and to Sarah Rubio and Debbie King for walking this road with me.

To my earliest readers and editors—Ann Swindell, Sarah Kelley, Stephanie Heilman, Erin Worrall, Shannon Williams, and Adrienne Garrison: Your fingerprints are all over this book, and you have each shaped it for the better.

To all the women mentioned in this book: I'm so glad our lives over-lapped during this sweet moment in time. Thank you for graciously allowing me to share your stories.

To Erin Worrall: You have made me a sharper, more self-aware, and more gracious version of myself. I say it all the time because it's unequiv-ocally true: I could not do motherhood without you. Thank you for all the times you've answered my exasperated texts, celebrated or cried with me, and helped me make sense of this disorienting season. But mostly, thank you for being my person.

To Dan: You believed in this book before I did, and you encouraged me to keep taking small steps toward it when I questioned my own ambition and ability. You were certain I should move forward even when the timing felt crazy, and you bent over backward to make sure I had the time not just to write a book but to write the best one I could. For so many reasons, this book would not exist without you, and I could never say thank you enough. You are the best thing that almost didn't happen to me, and I feel embarrassingly lucky to have you as my partner. What a life we've built. I love you forever.

To Selah, my first baby: You made me a mother, and I will never get over the joy and wonder of holding you for the first time. You are everything I wish I had the courage to be: expressive, silly, unashamed, resolute, spunky. Thank you for teaching me to take up all the space I need in the world. May you only ever grow bigger and bolder. I love you, precious girl.

acknowledgments

To Eamon, my rainbow baby: You redeemed so many sources of pain, both physical and emotional, and your birth gave me hope that healing is possible even when it isn't linear. When you smile at me, I feel like the most adored woman in the world. You have your daddy's eyes and my old soul, and I can't wait to discover more of who you are. I love you, sweet boy.

To Mom: So much of what I know about motherhood I learned from you. Thank you for every book you read to me, every notebook you bought for me, every imaginary game you played with me. Thank you also for the countless hours of babysitting you provided so I could write this book and for taking as much delight in my children as I do. You're an amazing mom, but I'm pretty sure you were made to be Gramma.

To Ken and Sharon Bergman: Thank you for encouraging me at every step, for believing in me, and for raising a son who would become an incredible husband and father. Our family life is richer because of your love and support.

To my siblings, Colin and Maddie: You were my constants in a childhood when we were always on the move. Thank you for being my faithful (and funny) companions then and now.

To you, reader and now friend: I'm so honored that you picked up this book and gave it your time and attention. Thank you for every essay you've read and every thoughtful comment you've left over the years. Your love gave me the courage to pursue this dream.

And finally to God—Mother, Father, Creator, Author: There are not enough names to capture who you are, not enough images to illustrate your goodness. You are even more loving and expansive than I dared to hope.